D1414897

Privatization and Mental Health Care

Privatization and Mental Health Care

A FRAGILE BALANCE

ROBERT A. DORWART and
SHERRIE S. EPSTEIN

Foreword by Leon Eisenberg

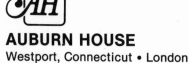

AUBURN HOUSE
Westport, Connecticut • London

Library of Congress Cataloging-in-Publication Data

Dorwart, Robert A.
    Privatization and mental health care : a fragile balance / Robert
A. Dorwart and Sherrie S. Epstein : foreword by Leon Eisenberg.
        p. cm.
    Includes bibliographical references and index.
    ISBN 0–86569–002–2
    1. Mental health policy—United States.   2. Mental health
services—United States—Finance.   I. Epstein, Sherrie S.
II. Title.
RA790.6.D67   1993
362.2'0973—dc20   92–38615

British Library Cataloguing in Publication Data is available.

Library of Congress Catalog Card Number: 92–38615
ISBN: 0–86569–002–2

First published in 1993

Auburn House, 88 Post Road West, Westport, CT 06881
An imprint of Greenwood Publishing Group, Inc.

Printed in the United States of America

The paper used in this book complies with the
Permanent Paper Standard issued by the National
Information Standards Organization (Z39.48–1984).

10 9 8 7 6 5 4 3 2 1

Copyright Acknowledgment

The authors and publisher gratefully acknowledge permission to use excerpts from: Dorwart RA,
Epstein SS. Issues in psychiatric hospital care. *Current Opinion Psychiatry* 4: 789–93, 1991.

Contents

Foreword

All mental health professionals owe a debt of gratitude to Bob Dorwart and Sherrie Epstein for this splendid monograph; it pulls together in a succinct and masterful fashion what is known and not known about the effects of privatization on the delivery of mental health services and analyzes the current state of affairs in a sober and thoughtful fashion. Dorwart and Epstein make clear that the field is long on claims for or against one or another position and disappointingly short on data to validate those claims. The data Bob Dorwart and his colleagues have gathered in studies carried out in Massachusetts and in a major NIMH-supported national study is about the best information available. Reviewing the available literature, the message the authors leave with us is the urgent need for systematic research on the outcomes of system-wide policy changes before state or federal officials buy into schemes, which are sold on the ground they will improve access but may instead beggar public providers (Clark and Dorwart, 1992).

Discussion of health policy faces a serious built-in hazard. On the one hand, the problems policy proposals attempt to engage are of daunting complexity; on the other hand, the ground rules for public debate allow so little time and space for presentation and rebuttal that all participants resort to evocative slogans that imply all-encompassing panaceas. Yet, at best, proposals must be provisional, in need of modification on the basis of experience after the policy has passed the point of no return.

Professor Michael Shepherd (1989) has reminded us that the danger was recognized in a remarkably prescient article on community mental health by the late Richard Titmuss (1961), the distinguished British sociologist. In the early days of the movement to return the mentally ill to the community, he pointed out that the pious hope so humanely expressed in the slogan of the movement (community care) could be all too readily mistaken for a reality that had not and may not be created. In his words:

It has been one of the more interesting characteristics of the English in recent years to employ idealistic terms to describe certain branches of public policy. The motives are no doubt well intentioned, the terms so used express, in civilised phrases, the collective aspirations of those who aim to better the human condition. It is necessary to remember, however, that this practice can have unfortunate consequences. Public opinion—in which I include political opinion—may be misled or confused. If English social history is any guide, confusion has often been the mother of complacency. In the public mind, the aspirations of reformers are transmuted, by the touch of a phrase, into hard-worn reality. What some hope will one day exist is suddenly thought by many to exist already.

Although Titmuss attributed the use of idealistic terms to "an interesting characteristic" of English social history, Americans have strong grounds to reject his chauvinism, I regret to say. When it comes to mistaking "the aspirations of reformers" for a reality not yet in existence, Americans can claim pride of place. Eminent Americans, including the presidents of Yale and Harvard, welcomed the promise of phrenology when it was introduced into the United States in the early 19th century. Phrenologists claimed to be able to read the features of the brain surface anatomy by palpating the overlying skull. This enabled them, they said, to diagnose strong and weak psychological "faculties," each represented in a separate anatomical area. This diagnosis then permitted them to design an educational program to strengthen the underdeveloped traits as well as to curb those that were hypertrophied. The claim of bettering the state of man made the movement irresistible to laymen and professionals alike in a country of boundless optimism. Some decades passed before the idleness of the claims became so evident that the movement was relegated to the circus sideshows (Davies, 1955).

A touching readiness to believe that American medical care could reverse the poor results of mental asylums in Europe permitted the rise of the "cult of curability" in the 1830s. Mental hospital superintendents employed year-end admission and discharge data to "demonstrate" high rates of cure (in one instance, a rate better than 100%) by such maneuvers as not counting deaths in hospital, counting as cured several times within one year patients with multiple discharges and admissions, and similar arithmetic sleight of hand. It was not until the work of Dr. Pliny Earle,

Superintendent of Northampton State Hospital (Massachusetts) in 1887 that the record was set straight (Deutsch, 1949). In a similar fashion at the turn of this century, in the early years of the mental hygiene movement, its evangelists promised the virtual eradication of mental illness through education in human relationships. Despite the noble motives and well-intentioned efforts, the millenium failed to arrive. The goals of prevention are today more modest but also more solidly grounded (Eisenberg, 1992).

Mistaking promises for reality remains a particular affliction of mental health policy pronouncements. In the mid 1950s and the years thereafter, "community mental health" was touted as *the* remedy for mental illness. Its earliest years were, in fact, associated with impressive gains; needlessly institutionalized patients (who had not been in hospital so long that their homes—and neighborhoods—no longer existed) were enabled to resume lives out of hospital. The reduction in inpatient occupancy was so rapid as to seem miraculous. Only later did enthusiasts learn how much of the decline represented transinstitutionalization (from mental hospital to nursing home) rather than the deinstitutionalization of long term and elderly patients. What stoked the process was the transfer of costs from state to federal budgets rather than the professed goal of humane care.

In his 1961 article, Titmuss anticipated the consequences of substituting slogans for reality in mental health services during the last two decades: chronically mentally ill persons discharged without appropriate provision for housing, clothes, and food, let alone mental health care. In his words:

To scatter the mentally ill in the community before we have made adequate provision for them is not a solution; in the long run not even for HM Treasury. Considered only in financial terms, any savings from fewer hospital in-patients might well be offset several times by more expenditure on the police forces, on prisons and probation officers, more unemployment benefit masquerading as sickness benefit, more expenditure on drugs, more research to find out why crime is increasing. At present we are drifting into a situation in which, by shifting the emphasis from the institution to the community—a trend which, in principle and with qualification, we all applaud—we are transferring the care of the mentally ill from trained staff to untrained or ill equipped staff or no staff at all.

Efforts to contain mental health budgets has led to a turning away from the public provision of services. The inability of community mental health centers (CMHCs) to solve the problem of the mentally ill homeless has led to blaming CHMCs for problems they cannot possibly solve in the absence of integrated housing, health, and social services. Today new promises are held forth. "Privatization" is the code word chosen to evoke images of efficiency, cost savings, and rapid response time. The "invisible hand" of the free market is to save us from "bloated," "selfserving" government bureaucrats. Little attention is given to the hazards associated with privatization: theft, risk-taking with public funds; pauperizing health workers; and unintended effects on the nonprofit and public sectors.

A December 1992 *New York Times* news account of a federal auditor's report stated that, "After years of effort to transfer government work to private companies, the White House acknowledged today that contractors are squandering vast sums . . . private companies had been paid for unauthorized and, at times, illegal expenses, including tickets to sporting events, lavish cruises and excessive salaries for executives" (Schneider, 1992). That report, I hasten to note, was not prepared for the incoming Clinton administration; it had been requested by the Reagan/Bush idealogues committed to the idea that private companies can do the federal government's work better and for less money.

The Savings and Loan (S & L) fiasco exemplifies the second danger. In this instance, deregulation made it possible to gamble with depositors' money at no risk to S & L corporate officers. Taxpayers are in the process of redeeming the resulting financial disaster. In the competition for mental health service contracts, there is equal reason to fear that low bidders will sacrifice quality of service. Moreover, as happened with several large Health Maintenance Organizations, low bidders may go bankrupt, leaving the community without services.

The third risk is to the mental health workers themselves. As poorly paid as are those in state employment, they have fringe benefits and some civil service protection against arbitrary dismissal. When their agencies are abolished and their jobs eliminated, they may be hired by the private contractor at lower wages and with neither civil service nor union protection.

The fourth hazard is that reinforcing the private sector may have major unintended consequences for the not-for-profit and public sectors in a health competitive-care market economy. The differences between the for-profit and not-for-profit sectors in health care are becoming vanishingly small as the administrators of the not-for-profits (who are, after all, hired to keep the organization from going into the red) shunt aside patients whose care is costly and reimbursement poor. Such patients are passed on to public hospitals, which find themselves unable to keep up with the rising tide of misfortune. A cascade of effects ricochets down the system.

I have, of course, revealed my own prejudices. What can happen is not necessarily what will happen. Some private services are excellent. Public

programs are themselves far from ideal. Many are inefficient, costly, and
of low quality. To repeat the words with which this commentary began:
claims are many, facts are few. What we can—and, I hope, will—agree on
is that privatization (like any other public policy) must be closely monitored. As the auditor's report to the White House noted (Schneider, 1992),
federal agencies "failed to supervise how hundreds of billions of dollars
are spent each year." That, in turn, resulted from administration decisions
to cut supervisory staff budgets. It suggested that "reliance on private
companies can only be effective if government closely supervises its
contracts."

Clearly, then, neither "community mental health" nor "privatization" is
a panacea for the problem of chronic mental illness. Whatever mix of
service patterns becomes public policy will require careful monitoring by
state and federal authorities. Precisely because their disabilities make it
difficult for severely ill patients to be their own advocates, there is a need
for close public oversight of the agencies designated to serve them.

Leon Eisenberg, M.D.
Professor of Social Medicine
Harvard University School of Medicine

REFERENCES

Clark RE, Dorwart RA. Competition and community mental health agencies.
    Health Politics Policy Law 17:517–40, 1992.

Davies JD. *Phrenology: Fad and Science*. New Haven: Yale University Press,
    1955.

Deutsch A. *The Mentally Ill in America, 2nd Ed.* New York: Columbia Univer-
    sity Press, 1949.

Eisenberg L. Child mental health in the Americas. *Bull Pan Am Health Organi-
    zation* 26:230–41, 1992.

Schneider K. U.S. admits waste in its contracts. *New York Times* December 2,
    1992, p. A–1.

Shepard M. Primary care with patients with mental disorder in the community.
    Br Med J 299:666–69, 1989.

Titmuss R. Community care—fact or fiction? In, *Trends in the Mental Health
    Services*. Freeman H, Farndale J (Eds). Oxford: Pergamon Press, 1963,
    221–25.

Preface

This book draws on nearly a decade of research by the authors conducted under the auspices of the Malcolm Wiener Center for Social Policy at the John F. Kennedy School of Government, and the Mental Health Policy Working Group in the Division of Health Policy Research and Education, both at Harvard. During this time, many groups and individuals have contributed significantly to various aspects of the research, and we wish to acknowledge their contributions and to express our gratitude. Indeed, we are indebted to so many individuals for assistance during this time, that it is not possible to mention them all nor to indicate fully the role of many.

The studies reported here were initiated in 1984 with support from the Division of Health Policy Research and Education and the Mental Health Policy Working Group. Over time, the three directors of the Division, Drs. David Hamburg, Julius Richmond, and Joseph Newhouse have generously supported our work. In addition, the directors of the Center for Social Policy at the Kennedy School, Drs. David Blumenthal, Mary Jo Bane, David Ellwood, and Julie Wilson provided valuable support and assistance. At various times, other Harvard faculty members (and visiting professors or fellows) affiliated with the Working Group provided advice and encouragement, including Professors Burton Weisbrod, Leon Eisenberg, the late Gerald Klerman, Miles Shore, Constance Horgan, and the late Manny Carballo. Several individuals contributed significantly as consultants to specific aspects of the research contained in this book: Drs. William Fisher, H. Steven Leff, Paul Cleary, Richard Pulice, and Robin

Clark. For his contribution as a mentor to our work as well as to the health of the public, we gratefully dedicate this book to Julius B. Richmond, M.D.

We wish also to acknowledge the advice and support of other members of the Mental Health Policy Working Group over the past several years: David Adler, Fred Altaffer, Paul Appelbaum, Jack Barchus, Arthur Barsky, Ellen Bassuk, Myron Belfer, David Blumenthal, Jonathan Borus, Stephen Buka, Jim Callahan, Hale Champion, Lee Chartock (Executive Officer), Stephen Day, Barbara Dickey, Glen Elliott, Mary Jane England, Shervert Frazier, Jon Gudeman, Philip Holzman, Robert Lawrence, H. Stephen Leff, Sue Levkoff, John Lichten, Benjamin Liptzin, Steven Matthysse, Thomas McGuire, David Mechanic, Martha Minow, Richard Mollica, Ann Moran, Evelyn Smith-Demille, Alan Stone, Ming Tsuang, Milton Weinstein, and Burton Weisbrod.

We were fortunate to have the support for various studies from the National Institute of Mental Health (NIMH) for a national study of psychiatric hospitals and for a Scientist Development Award to Dr. Dorwart. Additional support included grants from other sources for various aspects of our work, including the Henry Kaiser Family Foundation for work on this book. A number of people at the National Institute of Mental Health were very helpful in providing advice and technical assistance for our work, especially Paul Widem, Agnes Rupp, and the late Carl Taube.

A number of individuals served on advisory panels for this study and as reviewers or discussants of our work over the years. Data could not have been collected without the cooperation of several professional organizations, but especially the National Association of Private Psychiatric Hospitals, the National Council of Community Mental Health Centers and the American Psychiatric Association.

A special thanks goes to Mark Schlesinger, Associate Professor in the Department of Epidemiology and Public Health at Yale University, who collaborated closely in our work over the past ten years at the Kennedy School. His contributions as Associate Director of the Center and as co-investigator of research described in Chapters 4, 5, and 6 are gratefully acknowledged. He was co-author with us of many articles on related topics.

We have had excellent research staff contributions from many individuals in the collection and analysis of survey data, but especially from Harriet Davidson and Claudia Hoover. Numerous graduate students have participated as part-time research assistants on various aspects of our projects and we wish to acknowledge their enthusiastic assistance. Invaluable staff support was provided by: Kathleen Flynn, Corky Robinson, Mattie Hawkins, and Shelly Coulter.

Much of this book is comprised of original, unpublished material; however, because it is based on work we and colleagues have done over the past ten years, some sections previously have been published in other forms. For example, Chapter 3 is an abridged version of Dorwart, et al. (1992b), Dorwart and Epstein (1991), and Dorwart and Epstein (1992). Some of the ideas in Chapter 4 first appeared in Dorwart and Schlesinger (1988), Dorwart and Epstein (1991), and Dorwart, et al. (1992a). Portions of the results reported in Chapter 5 appeared in Dorwart, et al. (1991). The discussion in Chapter 6 is based on data that were presented in greater detail in a series of articles: Schlesinger, et al. (1986), Fisher, et al. (1991), Fisher, et al. (1992), Clark, et al. (1992), and Dorwart, et al. (1992a).

PART I

EVOLUTION OF MENTAL HEALTH CARE POLICY

CHAPTER 1 _____

Introduction

This book is about mental health policy in the United States, its evolution, current status, and future directions. We describe how the mental health care system in the United States came to work—or oftentimes not work—the way it does today. Mental health policy traditionally has been thought of as actions by government that result in programs on behalf of mentally ill persons. In the past, policies have led to treatment in state hospital systems, implementation of civil commitment laws, and the evolution of the community mental health center concept. Kiesler (1980, p.1066) has provided a comprehensive definition: "Mental health policy is the de facto or de jure aggregate of laws, practices, social structures, or actions occurring within our society, the intent of which is improved mental health of individuals or groups." Disciplines he identifies as involved in mental health care research and services include medicine, law, economics, epidemiology, and psychology. An excellent overview of these diverse topics is provided by Rochefort (1989). We focus in this book on current policy trends, especially those related to the economics of health care.

SYSTEM WITHIN SYSTEMS

A central thesis of this book is that the mental health care system must be viewed as a system within two other dominant systems: the health care and the social service systems. Indeed, mental health care overlaps to such a large extent with these other systems that it often appears to be a non-system, fragmented and inexplicably changing, reforming and reacting to external events. Rochefort (1988) sees both external and internal forces of change creating cycles of reform in mental health policies and practices. Viewing mental health as a subsystem has important implications not only for understanding how mental health institutions operate but also in determining appropriate levels of policy analysis. A good illustration of this approach to analyzing developments in the mental health care field is Paul Starr's (1982) analysis of the community mental health center (CMHC) movement. He places the CMHC movement in the context of the social program initiatives of the federal government in the 1960s, rather than viewing CMHCs as an innovation arising from developments within psychiatry. So, too, our approach places mental health policies in a larger societal context, wherein reforms internal to the mental health domain may have less effect on long-term outcomes than those without.

First, we review the historical background of the multilayered and fragmented mental health system which has its roots in earlier eras of social policy (Mechanic, 1989). The current system can best be understood in the context of these earlier attempts to form and reform mental health care (Morrissey and Goldman, 1984). Although approaches to treatment of mentally ill persons change from one era to another, basic attitudes and fears about mental illness may not. The long-term nature, heterogeneous expression, and poor outcomes of major mental illness treatment in the past account for much uncertainty on the part of the public and policymakers about what can or should be done in providing services. Acute medical care includes psychiatric treatments that involve drug therapy as well as other primary care medical services. Long-term care is given in state and county mental hospitals which provide "asylum" but may also be offered in residential homes and through home-care services. Criminal justice usually refers to prison mental health services but also may include "community protection" in a variety of forms. Social services connotes not only traditional social welfare services but also "case management" and educational functions directed toward patients, families, and the community. Critical to an analysis of these different care sectors is an understanding of contemporary financing and organization of services.

HEALTH CARE POLICY

The current public mental health treatment system in the United States has evolved in stages over the past century from one based on institutionalism to one based on pluralism of organizational settings and providers. Mental health policy has changed dramatically since World War II under the influence of three factors: scientific advances, social policy, and health care economics (Grob, 1987). Like health care policy generally, mental health care policy recently has been undergoing a series of major transitions, driven by the synergism of socioeconomic and scientific forces underlying recent "revolutions" in psychiatry: the introduction of scientifically based treatments such as drug therapy, deinstitutionalization of the mentally ill, and the expansion and commercialization of financing for psychiatric services (privatization). These developments have contributed in large measure to a "mainstreaming" of psychiatric services into health care as part of a process of integration of health and mental health services. Fuchs (1986) has identified four areas of integration in health policy which he believes must be addressed in the coming years and which are applicable to mental health care: inpatient/outpatient, physical health/mental health, personal health/public health, and the social services/health systems interface. Such dominant forces in health policy often drive mental health care in directions that may be beneficial to some patients but problematic for those with major psychiatric disorders.

Following World War II emphasis shifted from institutional treatments to community-based care. With the advent of federal funding, community mental health center programs developed throughout the country after 1963 (Foley and Sharfstein, 1983). There were more than 700 federally funded centers by the mid-1970s, and in 1990 there are more than 1,500 community mental health agencies identified by the National Council of Community Mental Health Centers. Some centers are large, others small; some are hospital-based, others free-standing; some treat many chronically mentally ill patients, others few; some are primarily government funded, others mostly privately financed. The centers were established initially through matching grants of federal funds that were intended to gradually decline so that they could eventually become self-supporting.

After 1981, when the mental health systems legislation enacted by the Carter administration was repealed in favor of a block grant plan, there began a period of emphasis on "privatization" in health care and mental health. Privatization denotes increasing reliance on the market and on competition for the provision of services by private sector providers. Some services are paid for out-of-pocket, some by third-party payers (private or public health insurance) and some through contractual arrangements wherein local and state governments purchase health and mental health services from the private sector.

The dramatic developments in recent decades in medical treatments available for major mental disorders helped make these private services possible, as institutional care was no longer the only option, and led to changes in the organization and financing policies of health care systems. Contemporary trends and forces from the general health care system include not only new medical therapies for mental illness but also diversification, specialization and expansion of the mental health professions, introduction of private and public health insurance plans, the growth of the for-profit hospital industry, and a shift from inpatient toward ambulatory care. One of the concomitants of these trends is the increasing tendency toward business-like approaches in providing health services. Medical care, and by extension psychiatric services, are increasingly viewed as "product" or commodity (Ginzberg, 1984). This tension between whether human services should be supplied because of a public obligation or mission to serve community interests or because of a desire to sell a service in order to generate a profit is one that we believe to be at the heart of many current policy debates in mental health. Pressures toward increased competition and cost containment are likely to exacerbate the stress already building as protagonists wrestle with various options for financing and organizing mental health care.

OUTLINE OF BOOK

In the early 1980s the Mental Health Policy Working Group at Harvard's John F. Kennedy School of Government conducted a series of studies on deinstitutionalization and other state mental health policy issues, such as the homelessness of the mentally ill, planning for hospital bed needs for the mentally ill, non-physician manpower and its impact on mental health care, and purchasing of mental health services by contract. Since 1985 the Working Group has focused increasingly on financing and organizational issues from a national perspective. With funding from the National Institute of Mental Health, we have undertaken studies on national trends and changes in the provision of mental health services in hospitals, community mental health centers and psychiatrists' professional practices.

These studies examine, for example, who is providing services, what services they are delivering, who is receiving care, and how the treatment process is monitored in hospitals and after patients are discharged. They also examine the effects on hospitals and other providers of factors such as ownership form of the mental health provider, competition, type of mental health facility, method of payment for mental health services and geographic setting for service provision. These studies suggest that the service system has changed dramatically in the post-deinstitutionalization era. There has been a rapid expansion of private hospital services, a fragmentation of community treatment programs, and a specialization of psychiatrist practice patterns. This reconfiguration of the service system is poorly understood and merits further study in planning for the future.

Part One of this book provides an introduction (Chapter 1), a brief historical overview of the development of mental health practices and policy (Chapter 2), followed by a review of recent trends and issues related to financing (Chapter 3). Part Two focuses on ownership of mental health facilities and how it affects those who need mental health services. Chapter 4 discusses privatization of mental health services. Chapter 5 summarizes our own studies with an emphasis on differences among public and private providers—the conflict of mission between health care as a commodity versus health care as a social good for the community—and the impact of competition on this balance. Chapter 6 discusses other studies, detailing the special problems for community mental health agencies and psychiatrists as privatization increases. In Part Three, we turn to a case study from which we derive policy implications and possible systems recommendations (Chapter 7) and conclude with a general political-economic analysis of mental health policy problems (Chapter 8). The concluding chapter also discusses how future policy may be directed toward improving mental health services by sustaining the fragile balance among competing forces and fostering a more integrated approach to providing care for severely mentally ill persons.

CHAPTER 2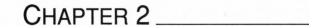

History of Mental Health Care Policies

INTERACTING THEORIES GOVERNING CARE

In this chapter we describe the four major theories and resulting methods of care that we believe have shaped the approach to treating the mentally ill in the United States. Although these methods developed chronologically, shaped both by new interpretations of what constituted mental illness and by evolving concepts of social responsibility, each method did not completely supersede another. Remnants of past views continued to interact with current ones, affecting and often impeding progress toward a coherent, stable mental health policy.

The first method, evident since antiquity, predominated in the colonial period: the mentally ill were treated as a deviant population afflicted by sin and in need of control by their communities; they were seen as little different from criminals who had to be confined and punished in repressive institutions. As the ideas of the Enlightenment spread to the United States from France and England late in the eighteenth century, many began to see the mentally ill as chronically ill and disabled, but not criminal or incurable; kind, humane treatment in retreats or "asylums" would benefit and even cure them. Although this second treatment theory led to a spread of such institutions for the mentally ill in the early 1800s, most of the disturbed population continued to be confined in jails and county poor farms. Significantly, even the enlightened physicians and public officials who thought the mentally ill would benefit from humane care believed they should receive that care away from society. When cures proved elusive, chronic cases accumulated in asylums in the last half of the nineteenth century.

As scientific medicine developed in the late nineteenth and early twentieth centuries, important findings affected the perception of mental illness. Most far-reaching was the chemical treatment for syphilis. With Salvarsan and, later, penicillin, most cases of syphilis could be cured, thus avoiding the end stages of syphilis that accounted for large numbers of demented patients in mental hospitals well into the twentieth century. Effective medical treatment for this pervasive condition led to a third theory of care in which mental disorders were viewed as acute diseases that could be conquered by modern medical discoveries.

At the same time, theories were developing that attributed mental illness to social and psychological causes. Sigmund Freud and Adolf Meyer in their different ways saw individual development, healthy and unhealthy, as the result of experiences in life and the effects of the social environment. The primary locus for mental illness has alternated between the physical and the psychological throughout the nineteenth and twentieth centuries (Rosen, 1968, p. 279).

The most recent theory is an outgrowth of the view that mental illness is a condition caused by failures of society. The neuroses or "shell shock" experienced by so many soldiers in World War I seemed irrefutable evidence that a biological explanation for mental illness was inadequate. Recognition that individuals functioned in a complex social structure led to the concept that mental illness could be prevented with the help of organized efforts in the community. Further, the community not only bore responsibility for causing the illness but for treating it; patients were not to be deprived of their civil rights or removed from their communities by confinement in often remote state institutions. This community responsibility theory resulted in the removal of the bulk of patients from state mental hospitals to be served by CMHCs in the latter half of the twentieth century.

We will explore the interactions of these dominant treatment methods over time as policymakers looked for solutions to recurring problems: how and where to care for those unable to function in society; who should be responsible for paying for their support and/or treatment; and how to balance society's need for safety and desire for orderliness with the civil rights of the mentally ill.

The Colonial Period and Social Restraint

During the colonial period in America, insane persons, especially those who had no family to look after them, were seen as dangerous and a menace to public safety; they were also nonproductive individuals who did not contribute to the community's economic well-being. Treatment of the mentally ill was consistent with the general practices that were common in Europe. In medieval times undesirables were banished, and this practice continued into the seventeenth century. But by the eighteenth, confinement of the poor, the unemployed, and the insane in almshouses became a novel solution throughout Europe that counteracted the effects of economic crises that had recurred since the fifteenth century. Unemployment and low wages had resulted in widespread begging and stealing, which was becoming untenable. Although there was some thought of improving the lot of those incarcerated, it took the form, as Foucault (1965, p. 47) explains, of preventing "mendicancy and idleness as the source of all disorders." Once confined, the unfortunates could be made to work and thus contribute to the community. Poverty and mental illness were not recognized as a fault of society, but as the outcome of an individual's vice and lack of moral behavior. By being willing to work, the inmates could demonstrate that they had conquered the moral laxness that had driven them to degradation. But the insane among the poor "distinguished themselves by their inability to work," and were punished for their idleness (Foucault, 1965, p. 58). The loss of reason was "an error to be rectified by disciplinary measures" (Rosen, 1968, p. 170). Adds Foucault, "Our philanthropy prefers to recognize the signs of benevolence toward sickness where there is only a condemnation of idleness" (Foucault, 1965, p. 46).

In America the colonists put the mentally ill who were thought to be threatening in jail, sent those who were not a menace but destitute to almshouses (usually farms), and banished those who were undesirable and transient from the town (Deutsch, 1949). Although the problem of caring for the mentally ill might demand a community response toward a dependent individual, the community's responsibility did not extend to nonresidents. Given the religious nature of a colonial community, and the then prevalent views about insanity, the town's response represented sanction toward an immoral member who must have sinned or been visited by the devil to have been so afflicted (Dain, 1964). Condemnation of those who didn't work was even stronger in America than in Europe. In this new land of opportunity, where labor was in demand, there seemed no excuse for poverty (Castel, et al., 1982).

The community's response to the mentally ill usually came from the action of the local overseer of the poor who was authorized to choose some arrangement for the care of the afflicted person (Lander, 1980). He might arrange to pay for boarding out, a form of foster care, in which private citizens were paid to board and care for insane persons in their homes. It was not uncommon, however, for the mentally ill to be auctioned to farmers whose care was contingent on hard labor. A less common practice was for the overseer to provide a home for the individual, paid for by the town or by charity from the church. The almshouse, however, was the principal form of poor relief in the American colonies in the late eighteenth century and provided shelter for the mentally ill on a larger scale than did any form of home care.

During this period we see the roots of subsequent public policies toward the mentally ill. First, there is the intermingling of public health problems with social welfare policies directed at poor and unproductive people in the community (Rosenkrantz, 1972). Second, there is a local, and later a state, governmental, or regulatory response that is largely administrative and organizational, focusing on setting policy to care for a group or class of people as a whole, with little regard for individual needs that might not respond to the approach chosen for the group. Third, there is the gradual emergence of social control through an institutional response in the form of jails, almshouses, and boarding in dwelling-care units (Rothman, 1971; Handlin, 1941). Fourth, there is a transition of responsibility from private means, such as the charities, largely religious, toward tax-supported government efforts (Grob, 1966). And fifth, there is recognition of the public responsibility to protect both society and the individuals from one another.

The implementation of these views worked unevenly then as now and resulted in widespread transiency, criminality, mismanagement, and inhumane conditions surrounding the mentally ill. These policies of social control continued to be influential as the public response to caring for the mentally ill turned toward building institutions designed exclusively for that purpose. The transition from the somewhat haphazard response of the colonial period to a more formalized one was gradual, and the change was brought about by several factors. Theories about the causes of mental illness were changing from the belief that mental illness arose out of idleness or sin to some understanding that any citizen and even kings (George III of England was an impressive example) could have strange mental afflictions leading to bizarre social behavior, caused presumably by some inborn defect (Dain, 1964). At the same time literature from Elizabethan times into the seventeenth century had been replete with characters driven mad by circumstance—Don Quixote, Lear, and Ophelia come to mind and there were many others (Rosen, 1968, p. 157). These examples illustrated a growing understanding that emotional and environmental factors and not supernatural ones were responsible for some derangements. Social problems were also becoming more complex. Growing industrialization and urbanization in the nineteenth century, along with increasing immigration and population spread in the United States, made it impossible for towns to sustain welfare functions by themselves.

The Institutional Era of Humanitarian Care

The growth of mental hospitals in the United States was a manifestation of the need for Americans to find a substitute for home and community to care for dependent members of a mobile society who could not live alone. The separation of the mentally ill from other dependents came about because influential community leaders had begun to believe that the needs of the mentally ill were different from those who were criminals or who were poor but sane.

A humanitarian approach toward organizing institutions for the mentally ill grew out of the Enlightenment of eighteenth century Europe and the writings of Philippe Pinel, the French physician who believed that removing restraints from "lunatics" and treating them kindly could effect cures. This recognition that the insane had rights to humane treatment followed the American and French societies' overthrow of tyranny and desire for liberty in the late 1700s. Benjamin Rush, the Quaker physician in Philadelphia, was the first to introduce kind treatment for mental patients in the new Republic, urging as early as 1789 that cells be heated and that brutal attendants be dismissed; he continued reforms over the next twenty years, publishing his findings in 1812, the first book in the United States on diseases of the mind and the only one until the 1880s. The old punitive correctional institutions for the insane were gradually discarded for new hospitals where treatment was decidedly more humane than in the past; the practices of using whips and chains were rejected, although bleeding, purging, and straight jackets were still used in many places when control seemed necessary.

The York Retreat in England, created by British merchant William Tuke in the 1790s, served as the model for hospitals built in the United States by American Quakers, who founded the Friends Asylum in Pennsylvania in 1817, the Bloomingdale Asylum (a part of New York Hospital) in 1821, and the Hartford Retreat in Connecticut in 1824. As described by the writers of that time, moral treatment was essentially social treatment rather than medical, based on what we would now term psychological principles; the aim was to create a family-like atmosphere (Bockoven, 1972). Education, recreation, rehabilitation in a religious atmosphere, and kindly interpersonal relationships would in theory bring about a gradual improvement or "cure" leading to discharge and return to home. The new concepts were accepted by prominent physicians in the large cities, but were probably little known to the vast majority of physicians who had not attended the country's few medical schools and were unlicensed practitioners in rural areas where there were no hospitals for the mentally ill.

Leaders of American society, interested in the new moral theories of treatment and influenced perhaps by those who believed at that time that mental illness was frequently found among the upper classes who had "superior intellectual talents," contributed to the founding of other private hospitals for the mentally ill such as the McLean Asylum in Boston (Dain, 1964, p. 35). Although some semblance of "public" hospital had been evident in the aims of the founders of the Public Hospital for the Insane in Williamsburg, Virginia in 1773, its financing was private. Not until 1833 was the moral treatment begun in private asylums extended to a publicly-funded one. In that year, under the leadership of trustees such as the educational reformer Horace Mann, who wanted to see these new ideas applied to a wider public, the Worcester State Lunatic Asylum in Massa-chusetts was founded. The need for something to replace the workhouse had also become apparent. Poorhouses had multiplied from 1821 on— Massachusetts, for example, had thirty-five in 1800 but more than one hundred by 1830—and nearly every state had them by 1830. Their function as workhouses had changed by the 1830s; Boston's House of Industry had become instead "a general infirmary—an asylum for the insane and a refuge for deserted children, the aged and infirm" (Deutsch, 1949, p. 129).

The Worcester Hospital soon became the model state institution in the United States. Its superintendent was the influential and well-respected Samuel Woodward, who administered the hospital from its start, coming there from experience at the Hartford Retreat. The hospital had been designed for 120 patients housed in small units, for it was thought that only in a small, personal, social environment could the moral treatment work effectively (Grob, 1966). Other states followed Massachusetts, and by 1844 eleven of the then existing twenty-six states had asylums and four states had two (McGovern, 1985). Unfortunately, the Worcester hospital was soon overwhelmed with several times the number of patients for which it was designed, and by 1850 it had at times over 500 patients. Overcrowding was typical in hospitals in the other states as well, and particularly bad in the South.

State legislatures "subordinated all other considerations in the interests of economy" and were content to build custodial facilities for the poor (Dain, 1964, p. 127). The state hospitals usually received funds from the patients' home counties and county officials were parsimonious in sup-porting the care of the mentally ill, often keeping them (especially chronic cases) in jails and poorhouses when possible because they cost less than the hospital. Funding for these state hospitals varied. Massachusetts, Ohio, and New York built them from state funds and had state officials administer them. Vermont's hospital was begun with a bequest from one person and finished by state funds; private subscriptions funded hospitals in other states. Cheap construction was usual, including that of the model Worcester institute (Deutsch, 1949).

Although Worcester and other hospitals had at first received lower middle class patients who could pay some fees, the majority of patients soon were chronically ill and indigent—a result both of state laws being passed to remove the mentally ill from jails and almshouses and the increasing number of mentally ill among the poor immigrants arriving in the United States. The population of the country nearly doubled between 1840 (17 million) and 1860 (31.5 million).

With the overcrowding of the hospitals came changes in treatment theories. Whereas in the 1840s, the superintendents of the mental hospitals had predicted that 90 percent of the patients could be cured and psychiatrists thought heredity could be overcome or its potential effects prevented by proper care, this optimism faded as their ability to administer personal, therapeutic treatment in asylums eroded. The moral treatment exemplified by the Quakers remained viable only in private hospitals where patients could afford to pay for it. By the 1860s, the poor mentally ill were being blamed by some superintendents for inheriting bad traits and accused of making their conditions worse by leading disorderly lives (Dain, 1964). More liberal physicians, however, like Woodward and Edward Jarvis, a leader in nineteenth century public health, blamed society for not providing good sanitation to prevent disease and for not educating people—especially those with family backgrounds of mental illness—in healthful living practices. Even these physicians, however, believed separate asylums for natives and immigrants were desirable (Jarvis, 1855).

It was soon obvious that there remained many mentally ill outside of hospitals and unable to receive care in the limited capacity of those facilities that existed. By 1860, twenty-eight of the thirty-three states had a state hospital for the insane, but the number of beds reached only 8,500 for a population of 31.5 million. In France at the time, there were 30,000 public beds for a comparable population (Castel, et al., 1982). The lack of a powerful central authority in the U.S., as contrasted with France, probably inhibited the growth of these public institutions since each state legislature had to be convinced of a need (Castel, et al., 1982).

In the 1840s Dorothea Dix, a member of the group of New England reformers and intellectuals interested in improving conditions for the poor, discovered to her alarm that there was widespread neglect and abuse of the mentally ill in Massachusetts. Expectations that humane treatment would reach those who needed care were not being realized and antiquated views and practices about treatment of the insane persisted. As recounted by Dix in her own voluminous writings (Dix, 1843) and by others (Deutsch, 1949), she found many mentally ill still in jails and poorhouses, locked in basements, and isolated on farms. Appalled by what she saw, she crusaded for expanded hospital facilities designed exclusively for the mentally ill, whom she said were sick people needing treatment, not criminals. She began by making demands of the Massachusetts legislature and then publicized her findings and extended her crusade to other states over a forty-year period. She has been credited with founding thirty hospitals. She advocated separate institutions for the mentally defective, the insane, and the criminal.

The Scientific Model: Madness as Illness

Well into the eighteenth century, medical treatment of illness of all kinds, including mental, had been based on erroneous beliefs that disease was caused by the interaction of four "humors." There was little or no knowledge of the need for cleanliness in preventing infection, and the skills of the physician were limited to bleeding and purging, usually doing harm rather than good, and the administration of a few useful drugs. Hospitals, poorhouses, and jails were little more than pest houses where disease spread rapidly. Charlatans with magic cures were common, flourishing in an atmosphere of ignorance and superstition. But in the eighteenth century the beginnings of modern medical knowledge emerged as individual men made important discoveries and society as a whole in the Age of Reason and Enlightenment began to be concerned with the care of the poor and the sick. The industrial revolution had begun in England and with it the crowding of the cities as people left their farms to work in the new factories. Deplorable conditions for the poor followed the crowding into dirty, smoke-filled towns (replicated later in the United States as industry spread to this country).

The advanced ideas of Ramazzini, a professor of medicine in Padua, presaged an understanding of the occupational hazards that had affected the workers in the factories as early as 1750. Glass makers, felt workers, and metal refiners were disabled—"mad as a hatter" was a commonplace simile—or died after inhaling fumes as they worked (Wain, 1970, p. 137). The Quaker physician, John Coakley Lettsom, published his findings in England about the addictive qualities of alcoholism in 1787, describing the effects of intemperance and serving eventually to separate, in some minds at least, madness from drunkenness. John Howard, a social reformer and sheriff in Bedford, England, became aware of the inhumane treatment of prisoners and reported to Parliament on the need for better sanitation and the separation of diseased prisoners from the rest in the late 1700s. Dr. Richard Mead, in 1720 London's most famous practitioner, realized that the plague was caused by something other than Divine Providence—he attributed it to "contamination of the air" and recommended isolating victims. With postmortem dissection, Giovanni Morgagni in Padua showed the anatomic changes brought about by disease and disproved the existence of "humors" in his publication on clinical pathology in 1761.

Although there was awareness of the existence of microscopic animals after Leuwenhock's invention of the microscope, it was still believed that they arose out of "spontaneous generation" well into the eighteenth century until it was disproved by Spallanzani in the late 1700s. Jenner's concept of immunity and vaccination came in 1800.

In the middle of the nineteenth century, as disillusion about moral treatment for insanity was setting in, the scientific knowledge accumulating began to explode into new and important discoveries. Antisepsis began with Semmelweis's findings in 1848 and Florence Nightingale's success with cleanliness in Crimean War hospitals in 1854. Virchow's concept of the body as made up of cells came in 1858, and Darwin's theory of genetics in 1859. From 1857 on, Pasteur carried Spallanzani's findings further, proving that bacteria could be controlled and leading to the antiseptic surgery of Joseph Lister in 1865 and Pasteur's own immunizations for anthrax and rabies in the 1880s. Robert Koch's improved laboratory techniques led to the discovery of a way to isolate specific microbes. In the years from 1880 to 1900 the causes of cholera, sleeping sickness, tuberculosis, diptheria, typhoid, tetanus, and dysentery would be found, and Koch realized that the flea carried bubonic plague.

A few years later, Paul Ehrlich, a pupil of Koch, was able to direct healing chemicals to specific bacilli. In 1909, after the 606th variation on an arsenic compound had been tried in animals, Ehrlich found the one that would kill the malaria trypanasome without killing the host animal as well; soon afterward he tried it successfully on the syphilis spirochete, recently isolated by others. His discovery, known as Salvarsan, proved too toxic to be the "magic bullet" Ehrlich thought he had found, but it pointed the way to better compounds and the possibility of cure. Syphilis in some form had probably existed throughout human history; a virulent outbreak spread throughout Europe in 1493, killing many; the minds of those who lived were often destroyed as the disease progressed, but the association of brain damage with syphilis was not made until the 1850s. In Germany in 1848 and 1851 doctors noticed that one-sixth of the patients in two different mental hospitals were paralytics and in 1874 a Danish physician showed that 90 percent of the paralytics in his study had had syphilis (Rosen, 1968, p. 255). The late effects of the disease, increasingly apparent as better living conditions and fewer cases of other infectious disease allowed people to live longer, would account for many of the inmates of the mental hospitals in Europe and America well into the twentieth century; indeed, Rosen claims that the general paresis (brain damage) resulting from syphilis "was one of the most common conditions among patients in mental hospitals" in the nineteenth and early twentieth centuries (Rosen, 1968, p. 279).

As these medical discoveries were being announced, psychiatrists found themselves disassociated from other physicians and disappointed with what they could accomplish with their patients. The crowding of the state hospitals with immigrants the doctors found hard to understand (literally and figuratively) made the intimate sympathetic help called for by moral treatment hard to achieve. Even in the private hospitals where moral treatment continued for a longer period, hope that these methods would cure mental illness began to fade by 1900. The realization that there seemed to be incurable cases—many with dementia associated with age or brain damage from the advanced stages of syphilis—even among the middle and upper classes turned psychiatrists away from a psychological explanation for mental illness and toward a somatic one (Dain, 1964).

The medical and scientific discoveries of the age showed that man could understand and control much that had been attributed to the will of God and influenced many frustrated psychiatrists to look for "medical" reasons for insanity. After Koch, they had some idea that lesions in the brain were the cause of insanity, but research was sketchy at best (Grob, 1983). At the same time, religion and morals were still strong influences and some psychiatrists continued to blame those patients whose behavior was outside the middle class mores of duty and work for causing their own insanity. By the end of the nineteenth century, institutional psychiatry represented the past and psychiatry was searching for a new approach (Grob, 1983). The institutions had become custodians again, relegating the mentally ill to a life apart, subject to a "legacy of chronicity" (Greenblatt, 1984). The accomplishments of the mental hospitals had fallen short of the hopes and expectations of the well-intentioned individuals who founded them.

Innovation came from outside the mental hospitals. The field of neurology had grown rapidly from 1874 on, and neurologists were critical of psychiatry as being "nonmedical." New terms arose, with "insanity" describing what went on in the asylums but "mental disease" used to describe a brain disorder to be treated medically by the neurologists (Castel, et al., 1982). Their research yielded little, however, and by 1910 there was a shift back to psychological explanations for mental disorders, ironically just as the medical approach was pointing to a cure for syphilis and its associated mental disorders. Nevertheless, the interest of the neurologists had made some long-lasting changes in the way mental patients were treated. General hospitals had begun to have psychiatric wards, some patients were seen in outpatient clinics, teaching and research on mental disease was conducted in major university centers, and the concept of follow-up services for discharged patients was introduced.

An important concomitant of the institutional period in mental health was the parallel growth of state bureaucracies that administered the mental hospitals and paved the way for the creation of state boards of health that would oversee public health and welfare programs. In Massachusetts, for example, the state had provided mental health services at the Worcester State Hospital since 1833, and Dr. Edward Jarvis had begun collecting statewide statistics on insanity in 1854; doctors such as Lemuel Shattuck and Henry Bowditch, as early as 1848, cited the state's involvement in taking care of the insane in arguing for extension of the state interest in other aspects of public health. They finally succeeded in forming a state Board of Health, Lunacy, and Charity in 1869.

The Progressive Era and the Mental Hygiene Period

The Progressive Era denotes a reform movement that began in the United States in the early twentieth century. After the Civil War, the industrial revolution that had transformed Europe came to the United States, and with it the factories and crowded, dirty city slums that had been common in Europe. Reform directed at improving the condition of the workers was led by middle-class women like Jane Addams in Chicago and Lillian Wald in New York City, who founded "settlement houses" that provided self-help programs for workers living in the slums. Other reformers attacked corruption in government and were responsible for legislation that brought about workmen's compensation, outlawed child labor, specified minimum wages, and introduced widows' pensions and maximum hours for work, especially for women. The Progressive Era saw enactment of the Pure Food and Drug Act in 1906, and an act regulating the railroads in the same year. Although the Progressives as a political party were unable to elect Theodore Roosevelt in 1912, the movement influenced enactment during the Wilson administration of the Federal Reserve Act (1913) and the Federal Trade Commission Act (1914); the Keating Owen Bill restricted child labor in 1916. After World War I the movement subsided and would not be revived until the need for further social welfare changes was seen in the 1930s.

As these social welfare rights were being asserted in the early 1900s, a gradual change in the philosophy and approach to the care of the mentally ill also occurred. Influential professionals like William James, Sigmund Freud, and Adolf Meyer aroused interest in the psychological processes that might cause mental illness; using their findings about mental processes and the motivations of the unconscious to prevent mental illness seemed to promise more than the use of moral treatment to effect a cure. At the same time, private individuals, most notably Clifford Beers, sought better treatment of mental patients, greater understanding about their disability among the public, and increased attention to prevention of mental illness through establishment of child health clinics. Beers, who as a young man had spent several years as a patient in public and private mental hospitals, became an effective advocate for better mental health services after publishing the story of his experiences in his book, *A Mind That Found Itself* (Beers, 1907). William James, a renowned Harvard philosopher and physician-psychologist, had been impressed with Beers and his manuscript and had helped him find a publisher. To launch his reform plan, Beers sought sponsorship from other eminent professionals, the most important of whom was Adolf Meyer. The Swiss-born neurologist-psychiatrist had worked at Worcester State Hospital and at Ward's Island in New York City and was at the time the most prominent hospital psychiatrist in the country. His appointment as professor of psychopathology at Cornell University Medical College gave him the opportunity to further his interest in combining research and clinical practice. His forceful personality and ability to influence his colleagues made him an effective sponsor; Meyer worked with Beers to found the reform movement sparked by Beers' book, usually referred to as the "mental hygiene" movement. Although other former mental patients had written exposés of institutional treatment, Beers' account was the most credible. It came from a Yale graduate who had been a businessman, it was well written and seemed authoritative. It voiced the perspective of the psychiatrists as well as that of the patient, thanks to Meyer's influence, and suggested reforms in a temperate manner. The book also came at a time when humanitarian reforms were the order of the day.

Beers spent the rest of his life on his reform effort and founded the National Committee for Mental Hygiene (later to be known as the National

Mental Health Association) to bring about cooperation between the health professionals and the concerned public, many of them former patients and their family members. No citizens' organization for mental health then existed, although some citizens' groups had been formed to found local health centers and settlement houses. The mental hygiene movement coincided with a recognition that public education about and intervention in the home conditions of patients was necessary; the profession of social work began around 1905 as these workers aided doctors and patients by investigating home conditions and educating family members in aftercare of patients. Beers' organization advocated that psychiatric hospitals be associated with medical schools to foster modern medical training and research in mental illness. It also advised the public on how to prevent mental illness, but has been criticized for expecting those living in poor socioeconomic conditions to be able to follow behaviors more achievable by the middle class.

The number of psychiatric patients seen in general hospitals rather than specialty institutions began to increase in the early 1900s as young psychiatrists found newly available teaching and clinical positions in university medical centers more attractive than work in state institutions. The criticism of state hospitals voiced by the mental hygiene movement, together with the influence of the neurobiologists who sought medical solutions for mental illness, resulted in an increase in patients seen in facilities other than state hospitals. The numbers remained small, however, and the bulk of mentally disturbed patients remained in the asylums because non-state hospitals were constricted in their ability to care for indigent patients. The private practice of psychiatry emerged in these early years of the century as the Austrian neurologist, Sigmund Freud, became renowned and his theories gradually gained acceptance. Freud and his disciples taught that unconscious drives existed and affected the mind, that childhood trauma was a cause of neurosis, and that the mind might repress experiences that later resulted in illness; they believed that analysis of a disturbed patient's experiences by a "psychoanalyst" could effect a cure (Levin, 1978). The first International Congress of Psychoanalysis was held in 1908.

These developments represented the beginning of a shift in emphasis from viewing mental illness as largely a public responsibility to one of seeing it as a private concern as well. (This shift would gain strength after World War II as the movement to privately insure against health costs eventually included insurance to cover mental health benefits.)

One aspect of the mental hygiene movement presaged the return to a community responsibility model in the care of the mentally ill. A critical theory held by mental hygiene advocates was that treatment of children's problems might prevent later mental disturbance. A clinic for juvenile delinquents was founded in Chicago in 1909 and an outpatient department at Boston Psychopathic Hospital studied children in 1912, as did one in Allentown, Pennsylvania a few years later. Traveling children's clinics were developed at the Children's Hospital in Boston in the 1920s. A team of consultants made up of a psychiatrist, a psychologist, and a social worker or a nurse would visit schools in surrounding towns to advise help for children who had demonstrated problems. A decade later (1932), twenty-seven large cities had full-time clinics for children and many more part-time child guidance clinics had been started (Rosen, 1968).

Post–World War I Period

Despite these stirrings, the first four decades of the twentieth century saw only a little progress or change in psychiatric care. Since state hospitals had become large custodial centers for the chronically mentally ill (including paralytics and senile aged), the mental hygiene reformers urged that other facilities be organized to respond to acute cases and to keep as many as possible out of the asylum. Emphasis would be on outpatient clinics, research, training of medical students, and follow-up care. Medical advances were changing the image of the general acute-care community hospitals as the new century began, making these hospitals increasingly acceptable to the middle class and not just to the poor who had no other options. Psychiatrists and neurologists sought to follow the medical model by forming "scientific" institutes known as "psychopathic hospitals" to carry out the aims of the reformers. Only about a dozen of these institutions, usually associated with universities, opened during this period, however—the first at Ann Arbor, Michigan in 1909—and they had little success in carrying out their designated mission. A major difficulty was the continued lack of effective methods to treat mental illness and the inability of the hospitals to return patients quickly to their communities. Rothman (1980) claims that the psychopathic hospital often served only as a brief first step to longer commitment elsewhere; both families and patients saw entry here as less stigmatized and more hopeful than admission to the state institution. These new hospitals thus became largely a place for diagnosis of the seriously ill, and treatment only of the relatively few whose conditions were likely to be short-lived and curable.

An important feature of one of these special hospitals, the Psychiatric Institute in New York, begun independently earlier but affiliated in the 1920s with Columbia University, was that the majority of patients were admitted voluntarily; most were young, and they were generally treated with psychotherapy paid for by families—hospitals like this one had little impact on the population that filled the state hospital. At that time, hospital insurance through Blue Cross, begun in the late 1920s, did not apply to private mental hospitals or cover mental illness since the state hospitals would presumably take care of such patients. Voluntary admission of the mentally ill to hospitals had been sought by mental hygiene reformers to speed up the onset of treatment and to equate mental illness with any other physical disability, but state hospitals had few such admissions. The state institution was increasingly known as a "hospital" rather than an "asylum" in the twentieth century as it sought to avoid the image of a totally custodial facility.

From 1922 to 1939 the makeup of the state hospitals remained roughly the same, with 13 percent of the wards occupied by senile, syphilitic, and alcoholic patients and 45 percent, by schizophrenics. More than half (54 percent) on a given day had been in the hospital for five or more years, and one-third had been there for ten years or more (Rothman, 1980, p. 350). Some 40 percent of the patients were aged 50 or more. It should be kept in mind that until 1935 the elderly had no social security, which might have helped maintain dysfunctional people out of an institution. Reflecting poverty and lack of other options, patients in the state hospitals continued to be over-represented by immigrants. In 1920 some 30 percent of the patients in state hospitals were foreign-born at a time when 14.5 percent of the U.S. population had been born elsewhere. Overcrowding was a problem in all the states. Between 1922 and 1939 the number of patients resident at any one time increased from 230,000 to 410,000, and the hospitals held on average some 10 percent over their rated capacity; by 1946 overcrowding would increase to 16 percent over capacity (Deutsch, 1949). By 1939, half the 130 state hospitals had between 1,500 and 3,000 patients, and one-fifth had up to 4,500 (Grob, 1983, p. 315).

The ratio of physicians to patients was very low, helping to fulfill the expectation that effective treatment was unlikely. Physicians could do little more than monitor new admissions for a short time; if there was no improvement, custodial caretakers took over. Problems in filling these staff positions were enormous; poor pay and long hours were compounded by little appreciation or diversity in tasks. Attendants seldom worked longer than four or five months; although most quit, many were also fired for drinking or for abusing the patients. Often the most long-lasting attendants were former inpatients who had trouble getting other work.

Despite these problems and the fact that the quality of care in the state hospitals varied considerably, overall some improvements had been made

by 1929 over conditions common in the nineteenth century. Fewer restraints were used; it was no longer usual treatment to give addictive
narcotics to pacify patients (although it still occurred); and patients were
separated by ward and sometimes by building according to the degree of
illness. Although the separation of patients was generally an improvement,
it sometimes became an excuse for control; patients who were seen as
uncooperative would be threatened with transfer to ominous-sounding
"back wards." Among the attendants in some places were nurses trained
in psychiatric care at schools in mental hospitals—however, half of the
twenty-three schools in the country were in New York State. Qualifications
for attendants were raised in some areas. Occupational therapy evolved
from having patients work at any sort of useful labor—usually farming—
to more individualized tasks, although Rothman claims that patients were
not taught anything likely to be useful outside the hospital. Hospitals were
concerned about abuse of patients and tried to prevent incidents. In the
decade of the economic depression (1930s), hospital standards, especially
for maintenance of the physical plants, fell as state budgets were cut, but
personnel, including psychiatrists, were easier to retain than they had been
earlier.

What happened to the specific aims of the mental hygiene reformers in
the period between the two wars? Where were the family care homes, the
outpatient clinics, and the aftercare they had recommended? Rothman
(1980, pp. 360–374) primarily blames the state hospital administrators for
wanting to retain their "best" patients to fill the hospitals' work quotas that
kept expenses down, but he and others also fault the lack of support by
legislatures, families, and people in the communities where out-of-hospital facilities would be located. Only a few states tried family care, or
boarding out, as a stepping-stone to self-support, and each program was
small. In 1939 some 1,300 patients were in family care at a time when the
institutional population exceeded 400,000. The reasons for the low number, according to mental health officials, included patients' reluctance to
leave the hospital and families' reluctance to take their own family
members home (despite fear of criticism for having someone else take care
of them in a family setting). Frequently the townspeople objected to former
patients living in their midst. Difficulty in finding suitable families willing
to board unrelated recovering patients was another problem. Also blocking
the innovation was the reluctance—often refusal—of state legislatures to
support anything over and above the state hospital, even if it might save
money in the long run. Administrating family care came from state hospital
budgets and state hospital personnel time. There was no incentive for
hospital administrators to encourage this.

Outpatient clinics were also administered by the state hospitals and suffered from the same problems in staffing and funding as did the family care homes. In the 1920s and 1930s the clinics operated by about half the existing 130 hospitals were open only sporadically—60 percent only once a month—and were ineffective. Whether hospital superintendents were convinced that only institutional care was valuable and outpatient care not worthwhile, as some claimed, or whether lack of funding was the main reason for avoiding any "extra" commitments, little was done. States like Massachusetts, New York, and Pennsylvania, which tried to administer outpatient clinics through their divisions of mental hygiene without resorting to state hospital personnel, were hampered by meager budgets during the Depression and they largely confined their efforts to founding clinics for children. Some privately-funded outpatient clinics—about 100—were in successful operation by the end of the 1930s. Follow-up procedures for patients who left hospitals were similarly sporadic and poorly staffed, with social workers in short supply to monitor the patients; there were, for example, five social workers to 2,300 patients at Boston State and four for 2,400 patients at Worcester State. The ratios were much worse outside of New England.

Psychiatrists, aware of the lack of progress in institutional care, looked for new methods of treatment that would not only benefit patients but would strengthen the profession's alliance with science and medicine, fields that continued to make important advances, e.g., isolating insulin to treat diabetics in 1922. In the late 1930s medical treatments for schizophrenics that employed insulin or metrazol, a drug that caused convulsions, became extremely popular, spreading rapidly until by 1940 almost every mental hospital was using them. This occurred even though there was no known physiological reason why shock therapy should work, proof of its efficacy was lacking, the mortality rate from insulin shock was 1 to 5 percent, and metrazol convulsions caused fractures. Many psychiatrists were critical of the procedures and use of metrazol was short-lived; it was replaced in 1940 by electroshock, which was easier to use and less dangerous.

The drive to find medical cures for brain disorders brought about the use of a radical treatment, the prefrontal lobotomy, that resulted in some 5,000 operations in the 1940s (Deutsch, 1949). Severing connections between the prefrontal areas and the rest of the brain altered personality irreversibly and the operation fell out of favor by the 1950s. Still another idea tried in the 1920s was fever therapy, directed at first to end-stage syphilitics since their paresis did not respond to Salvarsan. They were inoculated with tuberculin and mercury and eventually malaria-infected blood to induce fever, which seemed to improve their mental state somewhat. Experiments with fever therapy continued into the 1940s even though the process risked dangerous infections and evaluations of the methods were not subject to rigorous standards. Risky as all these procedures might be, they seemed to offer hope for improvement in patients where there had been none.

Some positive results of the search for medical cures occurred at this time. Pellagra, responsible for a small percentage of the psychotic patients in the hospitals, was found to be caused by a nutritional deficiency in the 1930s. The discovery led to a fruitless search for other nutritional causes of mental illness. The drug dilantin proved effective in control of epileptic seizures. After sleep induced by the drugs amytal and pentothal, formerly withdrawn patients became accessible to psychotherapy.

World War II and the Decline of the Public Hospital

Before World War II, more than two-thirds of U.S. psychiatrists practiced in public institutions (Grob, 1987). The accumulated dissatisfaction with institutional care, social policy initiatives begun during the Depression, the shock of wartime findings that indicated mental illness was more widespread than had been thought, and success in discovering drugs that meliorated the symptoms of mental illness precipitated a rapid change in psychiatric practices in the next two decades. By the 1960s, fewer than one-fifth of the psychiatrists in the United States were working in state hospitals (Rothman, 1980).

The need for government intervention to help distressed individuals during the downturn in the economy brought about social security legislation in the mid-1930s, aimed particularly at the elderly (many of whom were demented to some degree and were in mental institutions) and also aiding the retarded and other mentally ill. Insurance plans that spread the responsibility for paying medical bills to a wider public, rather than burdening only those who fell ill, had begun in the late 1920s. The early plans were tied to specific hospitals by the many Blue Cross nonprofit insurance companies. After World War II, commercial insurance companies with national capabilities began offering health insurance that covered all illnesses in all settings (McGuire, 1981). In the 1950s, experience with unexpected demand for psychiatric care distressed the commercial insurers, who then set maximum limits and demanded coinsurance payments for psychiatric care—a practice soon followed by Blue Cross—but there was now precedent for coverage of treatment of mental illness outside state hospitals.

Psychiatrists played an important role in World War II in screening recruits to the armed services and in treating those who broke down under the stress of war. Examinations designed to avoid recruitment of those subject to neuropsychiatric problems turned up a surprisingly high number of disturbed individuals among a young and presumably healthy population. Even though the examinations were criticized as unscientific and often cursory, the high number of questionable cases gave strength later to the arguments of those who claimed that greater attention should be paid to preventing exacerbation of as-yet mild mental problems among the general public (Lewis, 1948; Stevenson, 1946; Menninger, 1947). Grob points out that concern with the incidence of mental illness in the general population "represented an extraordinary intellectual leap" from looking only at institutional populations (Grob, 1987, p. 417). The documentation of the effects of prolonged stress on soldiers during wartime, who had previously shown no evidence of mental illness, would lead later to greater attention than in the past to social and environmental factors in the development of neuroses (Felix and Bowers, 1948; Grinker and Spiegel, 1945); mental illness was no longer attributed only to a failure in the makeup of a patient's personality. Success in returning soldiers to combat after brief treatment at local aid stations would lead later to the theory that prompt treatment in the nearby community was preferable to treatment in a remote institution (Grob, 1987).

After a dozen years of a depressed economy and four years under the stress of war, the health of the nation was perceived to be at low ebb in 1946. Interest in medical research and in reviving the lapsed physical plants of the hospitals brought legislation designed to build hospitals where they were needed most and to expand the formerly small and poorly funded National Institute of Health (NIH) in Bethesda, Maryland, the research arm of the Public Health Service. It had been necessary to carry out medical research during the war in nongovernment laboratories and now the government institutionalized this practice by having the NIH award grants to researchers in medical schools and universities under the guidance of panels of well-known scientists. Following this pattern, leaders in mental health care succeeded in convincing Congress to pass the National Mental Health Act in 1946 and to establish the National Institute of Mental Health (NIMH) a few years later. The new institute would award grants-in-aid for research and training, and for the establishment of mental health programs throughout the country. The hope was that early identification of problems would prevent serious mental illness and that the large state hospitals would be a thing of the past. The institute also funded study into the cause and treatment of mental disturbances; clinical trials of drugs that affected chemical receptors in the brain began to be carried out.

New exposés of scandalous conditions in the state mental hospitals came at this time. A liberal newspaper, *PM*, published journalist Alfred Deutsch's articles decrying conditions in the hospitals in 1946, which were published as a book, *The Shame of the States* (1948). The articles evolved from his history of the mentally ill published in several editions, beginning in 1937 (Deutsch, 1949). Mary Jane Ward (1946) wrote *The Snake Pit*, a graphic account of her incarceration in a state hospital; her criticism was further disseminated as a successful movie in 1948. As these influences converged to change the approach to combating mental illness, a significant breakthrough in medical research occurred in the 1950s; clinical trials proved the efficacy of the phenothiazines, antipsychotic drugs that controlled and mitigated the effects of psychosis, even in schizophrenic patients. Patients who could be maintained on the drugs were now able to function outside the hospitals.

These developments leading to treatment of mental illness in the community were accelerated by the social policy and civil rights agendas of the 1960s. Although the United States did not join other Western countries in adopting a national health plan after the war, vigorous discussion of it took place and by the time of the Johnson administration's "Great Society," consensus had been reached that the poor and the elderly should have government-sponsored health care coverage. Social security was expanded to cover most of the health needs of all the elderly under Medicare and of various categories of the poor, tied to welfare requirements in the states, under Medicaid. The many poor elderly who were in mental hospitals because they were senile or otherwise disabled and had nowhere else to go would now be paid for by Medicaid if they could be cared for in nursing homes. State administrators, eager to save money—e.g., one third of the annual budget of New York State went to care of the mentally ill in the late 1950s (Grob, 1987, p. 428)—moved patients out of the state hospitals and into nursing homes where the federal government would share the cost. Medicaid is funded by a federal/state partnership, with the state's share dependent on the wealth of the state. In 1963 nearly one-half (48 percent) of those who were categorized as mentally ill and over age 65 were in state hospitals, and the rest were in nursing homes. By 1969, these percentages had shifted significantly, with only 25 percent in state hospitals and 75 percent in nursing homes.

The civil rights activity of the 1960s that sought equal rights for blacks and for women extended to the mentally ill. The public objected to hospitalization of patients against their will in unsatisfactory facilities. The population in state hospitals had reached some 560,000 in 1955, and the Group for Advancement of Psychiatry (GAP) Hospital Committee Reports a few years earlier (GAP, 1948, 1949) had called for 300,000 more beds, but the numbers declined rapidly in the ensuing decades. Federally-funded community mental health centers (CMHCs) were established in 1963 and, as the state hospitals reduced their census, these new entities and the psychiatric wards in general hospitals increased their care of patients with mental problems. As the length of hospitalization was reduced (both through changes in theories of care and with the aid of the new drugs), private health insurers became more willing to cover hospital expense for mental illness, further reducing the need for state facilities. Treatment in non-state hospitals also made possible the care of many who had mental health problems but would not have entered a public hospital.

Community Mental Health Centers

Although the concept of community mental health centers (CMHCs) was one of the many developments resulting from changes in social policies in the 1950s and 1960s, as mentioned earlier, its more specific beginnings can be seen in the joint conference on mental health held by the American Medical Association (AMA) and the American Psychiatric Association (APA) in 1953. The conference called for a national report to set standards for future treatment of people with mental illness. In February 1955 Congress unanimously agreed to sponsor a study on the human and economic problems of the mentally ill and to fund demonstration projects on improving mental health services.

The study was carried out by the Joint Commission on Mental Illness and Health (JCMIH), a nonprofit corporation formed by the AMA and the APA, and financed partly by the pharmaceutical company, Smith Kline French. Its executive director was Dr. Jack Ewalt and the trustees were representatives of the professional societies of psychologists, social workers, hospitals, nurses, teachers, and other interested organizations such as the American Legion, the largest veterans' organization. The study report, *Action for Mental Health*, issued in 1961, strongly influenced mental health professionals and through them, the Congress (JCMIH, 1961).

Its recommendations were cited repeatedly in testimony before Congressional committees considering legislation aimed at helping the mentally ill, but its suggestions for rebuilding the state mental hospitals to establish hospitals no larger than 1,000 beds for chronic care were not emphasized by policymakers like Dr. Robert Felix, former head of the Division of Mental Hygiene of the U.S. Public Health Service, who became the first director of the National Institute of Mental Health in 1949. He agreed with and urged Congress to accept the sections of the report that urged expansion of local services (Grob, 1991). Professional opinion was that state hospitals had failed, and that community-based help for the mentally ill could be effective and more humane than that given in the hospitals. This idea, Grob claims, had not been well tested and there was no real basis for thinking that aid in the community would be successful, especially for the seriously disturbed population.

Among the report's controversial recommendations was one that proposed lay counselors rather than psychotherapists be allowed to treat "minor disorders," acknowledging that clergy and teachers were already doing this for many people; the idea was unpopular with those who embraced a medical model of mental illness. The chronic care hospitals proposed in the report were viewed by critics as likely to become second-class institutions to which patients would be relegated, perhaps in error, because predicting who would remain chronic and who might respond to treatment often defied existing expertise. "Action" called for a mental health clinic for every 50,000 in the population and a psychiatric unit in every general hospital of 100 or more beds—recommendations thought to be impractical by many. The report favored federal financing of mental health treatment.

The report went to Congress a few days before John F. Kennedy took office. Kennedy appointed a task force to consider legislation for mental illness and retardation; its findings resulted in a message to Congress from the President on the causes and proposed treatment of mental problems on February 5, 1963—the first time the subject had been given such prominence. His message emphasized poverty as an environmental cause of mental illness and called for preventive programs. Kennedy set a goal of halving the state hospital population in ten years. Going beyond possibilities suggested by the JCMIH, Kennedy saw patients moving from one service to another as their needs changed, all within the same community.

The Senate and House held committee hearings in the next few months as they considered legislation to establish community mental health centers. Senator Lister Hill's Committee on Labor and Public Welfare was convinced by mental health leaders that CMHCs were the answer to the problem, but hearings in the House raised questions. Representative Paul Rogers, knowledgeable about health issues, wondered where the personnel would be found to staff all the 2,000 projected centers. Others worried that if "temporary" federal funds were voted to staff the centers there would be pressure to continue such funding indefinitely. Details about the administrative methods envisioned to give continuity of care to severely ill people were not discussed. Eventually Hill combined two bills—one directed at the mentally ill and the other at those affected by mental retardation, a special interest of the President, whose sister was afflicted— and the bill was signed on October 31, 1963. There was insufficient support in the House for federal funding of staffing requirements and the bill went through without it (Foley, 1975). The legislation was officially called the Mental Retardation and CMHC Construction Act.

The concept behind the act was that a comprehensive community agency would provide a broad range of services to all who needed them within a designated catchment area of 75,000 to 200,000 persons. (This would later complicate administration of CMHCs in large cities where the catchment area exceeded these numbers.) Five essential services were to be offered: inpatient care, outpatient services, partial hospitalization, education, and consultation. The CMHC was not supposed to select its clientele by prognosis of illness, age, race, or ability to pay. Funding the agencies was an issue from the start. When proposed, the CMHC was to be a partnership of federal, state, and local governments, but as Levine points out, local governments have never been happy to pay for welfare and mental hospital costs (Levine, 1981). The act's authorization of construction funds only was soon seen to be inadequate and in 1965, despite the AMA's opposition, Congress authorized grants for staffing the agencies. The legislation allowed the National Institute of Mental Health (NIMH) to deal directly with local sponsors of the CMHCs. Stanley F. Yolles, the acting director of the NIMH, had favored direct funding to communities, rather than to the states, and his ideas prevailed, perhaps because the governors of the states did not object to this method of funding during Congressional committee hearings. Allowing federal funds to bypass the state governments was something entirely new, Grob asserts, "which inadvertently tended to diminish the authority and policymaking role of state governments" (Grob, 1991, p. 235).

The funding by the federal government was, however, a compromise between those who wanted no strings attached and those, like Anthony Celebrezze, then Secretary of Health, Education and Welfare (HEW), who objected to permanent subsidies. In 1967, federal support to operate the centers was promised at 75 percent to start but declining over five years, after which its share would be limited to 30 percent for a total of eight years. Celebrezze wanted federal money to spur new ideas, but thought local areas should be responsible for health care. The eight-year limit would allow funding of new centers as established ones began paying their own way.

The decision to fund CMHCs directly probably influenced those directing the agencies to view their mission as something other than care of the
chronically mentally ill; state hospitals remained in existence for that
function, paid for predominantly by state government. An even greater
influence in shaping the role of the CMHC, however, was the decision that
centers must eventually become financially self-supporting. Centers that
wished to flourish and sustain themselves after the termination of federal
support had to develop reimbursable (e.g., outpatient) services designed
to meet the needs of clients with some form of insurance coverage.
CMHCs would be criticized later for not treating the most seriously ill
patients who seldom had sufficient insurance, but catering their services
instead to paying patients who might have obtained treatment elsewhere
from private providers (Chu and Trotter, 1974). It is difficult to see how
they might have avoided this outcome, given the financing arrangement
legislated. Services important to the original concept, such as consultation,
education, and home visits, often had to be relinquished once federal
support ended (Woy, et al., 1981).

The provisions of the act had been vague, as is often the case with such
legislation, and implementation was left to HEW officials. Robert Felix,
by then in the NIMH, was the most influential official; his view of the new
act was that it would expand the aims set out by the National Mental Health
Act that had mandated research, training, and service; it would change the
way mental illness was treated, reducing the number of persons receiving
ineffectual custodial care (Felix, 1964).

The shortcomings of the new legislation were probably known to the
policymakers, but their efforts were concentrated on passing the legislation; solving the problems would come later (Grob, 1991). A major
difficulty lay in the assumption that patients had sympathetic families to
help them while they were being treated out of hospital—an assumption
disputed by an analysis in 1960 of the institutionalized population that
showed three-fourths had either never married, or were widowed or
divorced. The legislation did not make provision for or even discuss
housing in the community for those without supportive families. It did not
spell out how these new entities (CMHCs) would interact with the existing
mental hospitals, and although the act called for integration between the
CMHCs and medical hospitals, it did not specify how this was to be
accomplished. Specific staffing levels were not written into the legislation
even though inadequate staffing had been a recurrent complaint in evalu-
ating mental hospitals.

By the time regulations for the new act had been completed in April
1964, President Kennedy had been assassinated and his successor, Lyndon

Johnson, had begun his Great Society programs that called for money to be spent in other directions. In 1967 the war in Vietnam began to escalate and funding for CMHCs never reached the anticipated levels. Many communities could not support centers and in others trained staff was unavailable. The goal of 2,000 centers soon became unlikely. By 1967 only 200 centers had been built and, although Congress extended construction authority for two years and staffing for three in that year, the money appropriated was less than half the authorization.

It had been expected that funding to augment the federal input would come from third party insurance, fees from private patients, and state subsidies, but in areas where poor people predominated, these sources proved inadequate (Grob, 1991). The availability of health insurance payments depended upon having clients who came from a working population. Even when those who had mental problems were covered by an insurance plan, benefits were more limited for mental illness than for physical problems, and outpatient mental health care was subject to even greater restrictions than inpatient (Muszynski, et al., 1983).

The CMHC Act was being implemented at the same time that federal aid through Medicare and Medicaid and the Social Security Amendments to aid the disabled were passed (1965), all of which gave the state incentives to get patients out of mental hospitals where treatment was covered only minimally by these new federal programs. Medicare was designed as a medical insurance program geared to covering the cost of acute illness; only the medical management of chronic disease was paid for by the program. Medicare was enacted, too, at a time when mental illness was viewed as a chronic condition for which the state or local governments bore responsibility. Medicare policies established strict limits on allowable inpatient coverage for psychiatric treatment in specialty psychiatric hospitals and also restricted payment for outpatient services for the mentally ill. Coverage was less limited for general hospital care of the mentally ill. Medicaid funding, a joint federal-state medical aid program based on welfare eligibility, was not available for people of working ages (18–65) who were already receiving public aid by residing in public mental health facilities. Medicaid would, however, cover inpatient psychiatric care in general hospitals and in nursing homes.

As the new federal programs were instituted, effective psychotropic drugs were allowing shorter stays in mental hospitals. Together, these factors had begun to bring about a decline in the numbers in state mental hospitals before the CMHC movement had reached a level that would have accounted for the drop. Meanwhile, general hospital psychiatry began to play a significant role in treating the mentally ill.

The rapid deinstitutionalization that resulted in the late 1960s, at a time when there was little coordination between the state hospitals and the new centers, was a recipe for later trouble according to Levine (1981). The Department of Housing and Urban Development (HUD), which might have been expected to find housing for the mentally ill, had its own problems in securing funding and was unwilling to spend any of its hard-won funds in trying to house the mentally disabled who would have needed added assistance to live in housing developments; HUD almost never found funds to provide such help. A Comptroller General's study in 1977 discovered that only one HUD office had taken action to provide housing for the mentally ill by that date (Levine, 1981). The social security payments to the mentally disabled went to the individuals affected, but those who were resident in public institutions were not eligible to receive disability funds. As a result, to receive social security aid, many moved to substandard boarding homes or single rooms in hotels where they received no mental health services or professional supervision.

Locating suitable space for community mental health centers was another basic difficulty since other groups doing community service often competed for the same space in the center cities. CMHC clients were not welcomed even in poor neighborhoods. Attitudes toward the mentally ill had changed since the colonial period, but antagonism had not disappeared.

Congress continued to renew the CMHC Act from 1965 until 1970 and extended coverage in CMHCs to drug and alcohol abusers. In 1968 funding was provided to evaluate the effectiveness of CMHCs; the subject of community mental health services became a new professional specialty for researchers. The 1970 renewal of the act increased funds for children and extended staffing grants, as well as consultation and education funds. Requirements were modified to make the start-up of centers in poor areas easier to accomplish. In 1967 federal support had been given to 186 centers and by 1970 the number had grown to 450. Growth slowed after 1970, however, as the Nixon administration was unsympathetic to spending for research and training in mental health. In fact, Nixon impounded the funds that Congress had authorized for the program and the funds were not released until he was ordered to do so by the courts in 1973. By 1970 some communities were dropping the CMHC programs as federal support fell off when seed money was used up in the planned funding decline (Levine, 1981). By 1973 there were 492 federally-sponsored centers.

President Ford continued opposition; renewal of CMHC legislation was only passed over his veto in 1975. The amendments that year extended some funds to centers when their basic federal grants had expired, and called for additional services to the elderly, minorities, and rape victims. In that year only 507 centers were operating, although some others had received initial grants. By 1980 there were 691 CMHCs (Manderscheid, et al., 1984). About a third of them had completed their cycle of federal funding (Woy, et al., 1981). Annual federal expenditures for the program averaged about $200 million until 1975, but were reduced by nearly one-half after that. The lack of adequate federal support meant that centers had to rely on other sources; insurers, however, did not support programs formerly paid for by federal aid, such as halfway houses or day care or, in many cases, care by paraprofessionals. Total funds allocated by the federal government between 1966 and 1980 were $2.8 billion.

Poor coordination of fragmented services to the mentally ill remained a problem despite good intentions; Levine reports eleven federal departments and agencies responsible for 135 programs for the mentally ill in 1980 (Levine, 1981). The CMHC concept had not been as well carried out as had been hoped by the sponsors of the legislation. Without support services, the seriously mentally ill could not function out of hospitals; needed were supervised living arrangements, help with income, employment, medical care, education, and even recreation and transportation. The CMHC was unable to provide all of these or to coordinate programs that existed in separate agencies. The outcome of these difficulties was a continuing problem of housing the mentally ill, unsolved by 1990 (Levine and Rog, 1990; Carling, 1990).

In the 1980s the Reagan administration's policies of shifting responsibility for social programs to the states and away from the federal government resulted in much-reduced funding for CMHCs. The 1981 budget act instituted alcohol, drug abuse, and mental health block grants to the states, out of which CMHCs that had already been funded were to continue to receive money, but the level of funding was not specified. About a third of the block grant went to alcohol services, another third to drug abuse, and the rest to mental health, including CMHCs. The funding for all three services was reduced by 21 percent in 1982—more if inflation is considered. Not only were CMHCs affected by the varying capacities and desires of the states to augment diminished federal funds, but the lack of uniform data collection once the federal government relinquished responsibility meant that evaluation of the effects of block grants was carried out only episodically. One study that sampled thirty-six centers in eight states found that centers were battling staff reductions and were attempting to increase both the number of private paying patients and the amount of their charges to clients (Estes and Wood, 1984).

Despite the problems in financing and in treating the seriously ill, CMHCs have provided an alternative to hospital care for many with mental problems. Studies have shown that community services reduce the need for hospitalization or reduce the amount of recidivism by as much as half (Anthony, et al., 1972; Test and Stein, 1976; Gottesfeld, 1976). Community resources resulted in a shift in episodes of care from inpatient to outpatient (Windle, et al., 1974). Community visits carry less stigma than hospital admissions and, even when repeated visits are necessary, can help a patient cope with illness rather than try to avoid treatment (Beebe, 1990). Halfway houses sponsored by community services have been found to help some 80 percent of the residents (Rog and Rausch, 1975) and act as an informal resource for ex-residents who live nearby (Berman and Hoppe, 1976).

A Shift Toward Privatization

The Reagan administration's ADM (alcohol, drug, and mental health) block grants gradually came to be dominated over the 1980s by funds for combating drug abuse. The federal government continued to provide planning grants to states for community mental health services but virtually abandoned direct funding of services.

Medicare and Medicaid continued to finance psychiatric services; however, the particular restrictions on eligibility as to site of service, personal characteristics of beneficiaries, types of treatments and extent of coverage served to shape mental health care in the 1980s. As initially envisioned in the CMHC legislation and promoted under the Nixon administration, CMHCs began to shift away from government support. As private insurers and state governments followed the lead of federal policymakers, the era of privatization in the 1980s and 1990s began.

CHAPTER 3 _____

Financing of Mental Health Services

BACKGROUND: TRENDS IN MENTAL HEALTH CARE COSTS

As we have shown, prior to World War II, states assumed the primary financial responsibility for caring for the mentally ill. In 1946, the National Mental Health Act authorized federal expenditures for research, training of personnel, and assistance to states to develop new mental health programs. Federal support of mental health research increased during the next decade. Professional and citizen involvement helped shift the focus of care from long-term chronic care in often distant state hospitals to short-term inpatient care combined with outpatient care in the patients' own communities. This shift in focus culminated in 1963 with the passage of the Community Mental Health Centers Act.

As the definitions of mental illness became more medically oriented and the treatment methods changed, mental health care became by the 1950s—and increasingly so in the past few decades—a service covered also by health insurance, both public and private. The total direct costs of alcohol, drug abuse, and mental health care in the United States accounts,

Portions of this chapter were excerpted from our more comprehensive review of financing methods for mental health services published in *The Textbook of Administrative Psychiatry*, edited by JT Talbott, RE Hales, and SL Keill, issued by the American Psychiatric Press, Inc. in Washington, DC in 1992. We gratefully acknowledge the editors' permission to include that material here.

by most estimates, for nearly 15 percent of the more than $600 billion spent on health care in 1990 (APA, 1989). Not included in these estimates are the costs of social and legal services, and of lost employment among those who were ill, and among family caregivers.

Changing patterns of payment for services have fostered the shift from separate public and private systems of hospital care to a mixed public-private system in which hospitals of all types—specialty and general—increasingly rely on multiple sources of revenue. Financing arrangements have become diverse and complex. Today, only about a third of the mental health services are funded by non-market sources (largely public mental hospitals and the Veterans Administration) and the rest by market-oriented mechanisms (providers paid out-of-pocket or by private insurance or by public entitlement programs like Medicare or Medicaid) (McGuire, 1989a).

These changes in financing toward a more market-oriented situation have several effects. As competitive pressures on hospitals increase, there is reduced financial access for some patients as well as expanded options for others. Not only the uninsured patient but those seen as costly or difficult to treat are often viewed as less desirable to hospitals that must maintain a mix of revenues in order to make a profit or to survive financially.

Since the beginning of the community mental health center era in the 1960s, there has been a shift toward outpatient care for the mentally ill rather than care in hospitals and a greater reliance on services provided under the auspices of private providers rather than public sources (Dorwart and Schlesinger, 1988). Consistent with recent concern about rising health care costs and changes in health care financing generally, there has been of late an emphasis on new types of compensation for mental illness care, designed to hold down costs, such as prospective payment systems, market-based fee schedules (known also as relative value fee systems), and capitation plans. These changes have made financing of mental health care complicated and fragmented for providers and clients alike. For the severely mentally ill, the market model is especially difficult to negotiate.

Health care financing in this country was profoundly changed by the emergence of private health insurance in the 1930s. Insurance made it possible for many more Americans to pay fully for the medical care they needed and fueled a rapid expansion in the number and treatment capacity of providers. When health benefits were substituted for wage increases during World War II, they became an institutionalized and popular fringe benefit of employment, and in the following decades the majority of

Americans were receiving some type of insurance coverage for their medical bills.

It was at this point that competition first began to reshape the financing of health care. The first insurers were nonprofit groups (Blue Cross) regulated by the states whose premiums were based on "community rating," a system in which all resident, of a community were charged an average rate. As private for-profit insurers entered the market, this system gave way to "experience rated" policies with premiums based solely on the health care costs of more limited groups. By shifting to experience rating, an employer with young and relatively healthy employees could avoid paying the costs of older retirees who had higher health expenses. Though experience rating was financially attractive to employers and their employees, it had its cost for the society at large. Because the disabled or retired had high health care costs, a private insurance plan composed exclusively of these groups had extremely high premiums, well beyond what was affordable to most Americans. Indeed, it was in part the shift from community to experience rating that prompted the passage in 1965 of Medicare, a public insurance program with subsidized premiums for the elderly, and Medicaid, a public insurance plan for those on welfare. (See further discussion of these programs below.)

Health care costs have rapidly escalated over the past several decades. This has further focused our health care financing system on more narrowly-defined private interests. Health benefits now represent between 7 and 8 percent of employee compensation, and will reach 10 percent by the mid-1990s. To American employers increasingly concerned with international competition, this appears to be an ever-growing burden. Throughout the 1980s we have struggled to reduce the costs in two ways—by reducing the coverage of employer-subsidized policies and by paying less for care that is purchased under those policies.

To hold down costs, employers have sought to reduce the dollar amount or kind of coverage in their health insurance policies. The groups who bear the largest cutbacks are those who are least effectively represented in the negotiations—retired workers and dependents. In some cases, these cutbacks take the form of reductions in coverage of specific services for dependents, such as psychiatric care for adolescents. In other cases, the amount of employer payments for dependents' coverage may be reduced or eliminated entirely. This can make the cost of insurance for dependents beyond the means of many working Americans. As of 1985, for example, three million children who were uninsured lived in households where the working parent had insurance.

Employers' primary strategy for holding down medical costs, however, has been to negotiate lower prices with the physician groups or hospitals from which they are purchasing medical services. As with the earlier shift from community-rated to experience-rated insurance, this holds down costs to the employer. But again, the primary consequences are felt by those unable to pay for their own medical care. Discounted pricing squeezes down providers' profits from those who can pay for services, making them less able to subsidize the costs of those who lack insurance or other financial resources.

Providers' reduced ability to subsidize the care of the uninsured has been reinforced by their reduced willingness to view this as an important goal. This is reflected in the growth of corporately-owned health care facilities. Unlike nonprofits, they have no obligation to philanthropy or obligation to pay back in free care the contributions made by government in building their hospitals under the Hill-Burton Act passed after World War II. Profit-making providers tend to be oriented to the bottom line and unlikely to view treating unprofitable patients as part of their organizational mission. Investor-owned hospitals, for example, are three to five times as likely to discourage admissions by uninsured patients than are comparable hospitals operated by private nonprofit or public agencies. But similar practices have begun to emerge in nonprofit institutions as well.

In a time of public and private pressure to reduce health care costs and institutional capacity in the health care system generally, it is somewhat remarkable to observe this growth in private psychiatric hospital care. In our assessment, this growth is attributable in part to the very fact that mental health care in the United States is at a somewhat different evolutionary stage than much of the rest of health care. While general hospital care is marked by the increasing use of prospective payment by insurers and restrictions on insurance coverage, as well as by public and private policies designed to move patients from inpatient to outpatient settings, mental health care has been characterized by continued cost-based reimbursement, stable or expanding insurance coverage, and a perception that public policies may have pushed too far in the quest for deinstitutionalization. These differences in themselves may make mental health care a promising market for investors. But they also reflect three more complex and important ongoing trends that are critical determinants of the privatization of mental health care. These are continued growth of the demand for psychiatric hospital care, ongoing changes in the general health care system, and changes in the goals of state policymakers.

In this chapter, we describe the major elements of the health financing system as it applies to mental health care and substance abuse treatment

Figure 3.1
Expenditures by type of mental health organization, 1986.

	Expenditures (in billions)	Percent
Total	$18.5	100.0%
State and County Hospitals	6.3	34.0
Private psychiatric hospitals	2.6	14.0
Nonfederal general hospital psychiatric units	2.8	15.0
Veterans Administration	1.4	7.6
Community mental health centers	3.7	20.0
Residential treatment centers for children	1.0	5.4
Freestanding outpatient clinics	.5	2.7
Freestanding partial care psychiatric organizations	.07	0.3

Source: National Institute of Mental Health, Statistical Note No. 193, August 1990. DHHS Publication No. (ADM) 90–1699.

in both public and private sectors. We outline the role played by the federal government in paying for services. We review the financing responsibilities still held by state and local governments and the significant part played by insurance mechanisms and self pay in funding services. In addition, we discuss selectively some of the newer developments likely to influence the provision of care in the future, such as managed care, capitation, diagnosis-related groups, and the resource-based relative value scale. We discuss, as well, problems connected with financing care of mentally ill children and of people who abuse substances.

Overview of Expenditures: Public versus Private

Data available to show how money is spent on mental health care cover only the amount spent on organized mental health programs, making up what is known as specialty mental health. These data, collected by the federal government, do not include the expense of psychiatric care given by psychiatrists or other health practitioners in their offices. In 1986, expenditures for organization-based mental health were estimated at $18.5 billion (Sunshine, et al., 1990). The amount spent per capita has not varied appreciably since 1969 if inflation is taken into account, but there have been marked shifts in where the money was spent. A decline in the amount spent in the diminishing state and county mental hospitals was matched by increases spent on psychiatric services in general hospitals and in private psychiatric hospitals.

Expenditures by type of mental health organization in 1986 are shown in Figure 3.1 (Sunshine, et al., 1990). Although state and county mental hospitals continued to account for the bulk of expenses (34 percent) to cover the care of the most seriously ill, psychiatric units in short-term general hospitals were the most likely place for hospitalization for a mental disorder (Wallen, 1986). Expenditures for such treatment accounted for 15 percent of the total—about the same as the amount spent on private psychiatric hospitals. Expenditures for community mental health centers amounted to about 20 percent of the $18.5 billion total. The Veterans Administration, with some 10 percent of the psychiatric beds in the country, accounted for 7.5 percent of the expenditures.

The sources of funds for mental health services have to some extent determined where care is given. As private insurance to cover mental illness became more prevalent, private psychiatric hospitals, many of them for-profit, grew in number. Medicaid rules that did not allow payment to psychiatric hospitals for adults under 65 spurred the development of psychiatric units in general hospitals where treatment was paid for by the shared state/federal program. Overall, states continue to be the major source for payment to mental health specialty facilities. NIMH data (Sunshine, et al., 1990) show the distribution of revenue sources for 1986 as:

State funds (not Medicaid)	48.1%
Federal (not Medicare or Medicaid)	10.3
Medicaid*	9.0
Medicare	3.0
Local government	7.8
Patient fees (includes insurance)	16.7
Other	5.1

*Including federal and state shares.

Although local governments paid only a relatively small share of costs overall, they were especially important to free-standing psychiatric clinics serving outpatients and to community mental health centers where they provided about a fifth of revenues. Fees (including insurance) paid for the bulk of private psychiatric hospitals' total costs (67 percent), but only 10 to 15 percent of outpatient-oriented organizations' costs, and about 4 percent of the costs in state hospitals.

The federal government paid for all the substantial Veterans Administration mental health component, for Medicare, its share of Medicaid, and the block grants to the states for alcohol and drug abuse and mental health treatment. The federal government also funds the income supplement to social security (Supplementary Security Income or SSI), which, since 1974, has provided a basic monthly benefit to the disabled with no other sources of income who are not in an institution, and, since 1972, the disability insurance for those eligible under social security—people with a work history (Social Security Disability Insurance or SSDI). SSDI is paid for through Medicare, extended to those under 65 who are disabled. The public sector supplies the bulk of support and treatment for the severely mentally ill. An estimated one fourth of those receiving SSI are disabled by mental illness (Adams, et al., 1989). In 1988 the federal government spent $3.8 billion dollars for SSDI and $1.6 billion for SSI to support people with mental illness (Scallet, 1990). These large sums translate into widely varying individual benefits. States can supplement the SSI federal benefit level and the wealthier states do so, but the SSI benefit is generally below the federal poverty level or at best only slightly above it.

Medicaid is a major payor for mental health services. (SSI recipients are automatically enrolled in Medicaid.) In specialty facilities its 9 percent share of revenues accounted for $1.4 billion in 1986. Medicaid paid for a slightly higher percentage (11 percent) of state hospital costs. The Medicaid program is administered by the states, each of which determines funding levels and eligibility; the federal government provides about half the funds overall, but its share is higher in poor states. Medicaid historically has not paid for support services outside health facilities for the mentally ill living in the community—thus encouraging episodes of care in acute care facilities rather than ongoing supportive help in daily living. Medicaid is tied to eligibility for welfare but state programs vary so much that many people below the poverty line do not receive benefits and some who are above it do receive them.

Public Insurance

Medicare. The Medicare program was enacted in 1965 as Title XVIII
of the Social Security Act. It is a two-part health insurance program, partly
financed through a payroll tax and trust fund, available to all persons in
the U.S. over age 65 who are eligible for social security, and some disabled
persons under 65 years of age, including those with end-stage kidney
disease. Although disabled people under age 65 account for only 9.5
percent of the overall Medicare population, they use disproportionately
more mental health services. Approximately 11 percent of all Medicare
hospital discharges were from this disabled population, whereas about 39
percent of the Medicare discharges with a mental illness diagnosis were
disabled (Lave and Goldman, 1990).

Medicare covers hospital care, extended care, and some home health
services. Coverage for psychiatric patients is similar to coverage for other
important medical conditions except for one major distinction—a limitation on lifetime reserve for those in a psychiatric institution. Medicare
eligibles are automatically enrolled in Part A, which provides up to ninety
days of inpatient care in each benefit period, with each term of hospitalization to be broken by a sixty-day interval between benefit periods. A
sixty-day "lifetime reserve" can extend any benefit period. However, if a
patient is in a psychiatric "free standing" hospital rather than a general
hospital, coverage is limited to 190 days of care in a patient's lifetime and
may not be extended by the reserve. These limitations have helped to shift
psychiatric care to general hospitals.

Part B is a voluntary enrollment program for which the insured pays a
monthly premium; it covers 80 percent of allowable physician costs and
outpatient services. Enrollees are responsible for copaying the other 20
percent. Coverage for physician services for psychiatric patients in a
hospital setting is comparable to that for general health care. However,
until 1990, coverage for outpatient mental health services has been severely limited and not equal to that for general health services. The
Omnibus Reconciliation Act of 1987 expanded the covered limit to $2,200
from the $500 set in 1966, but retained a 50 percent coinsurance require-
ment. In 1989 the ceiling of $2,200 per year for outpatient services was
lifted in recognition of the medical nature of many disorders. Copayments
by the elderly have been 50 percent for outpatient mental health services,
in contrast to 20 percent for general health services. In 1990, however,
those visits designated for changing or monitoring psychiatric medication
were, for the first time, covered similarly to other health services and
copayment was reduced to 20 percent.

The Epidemiologic Catchment Area (ECA) study carried out in five cities in the early 1980s indicated that approximately 12.3 percent of those over age 65 have a diagnosable mental disorder (Regier, et al., 1988). They are less likely than those younger to seek treatment for these disorders, and much less likely to obtain care from specialty mental health providers (Shapiro, et al., 1984). In 1987, approximately 2.7 percent of Medicare payments were for alcohol, drug, and mental health services (Health Care Financing Administration, HCFA, data in Lave and Goldman, 1990). This allocation differs from private health insurance programs for which 7 to 18 percent of expenditures are for these services (Schlesinger, 1989). Outpatient mental health care is a very small portion of Medicare expenditures, amounting to less than 0.1 percent of total costs (McGuire, 1989b). There is concern that the small portion reflects an underuse of mental health services by Medicare beneficiaries (Lave and Goldman, 1990).

Medicaid. Medicaid, like Medicare, was enacted in 1965 and is a major source of financing of care for the indigent mentally ill. As Title XIX of the Social Security Act, its purpose is to help fund medical care for the poor by providing federal matching funds to the states. Depending on the wealth and policies of the state, the state's share of the total funding varies between 17 and 50 percent. Medicaid must provide health benefits to those people receiving Aid for Dependent Children (AFDC), the blind, the totally and permanently disabled, and low-income persons 65 years of age or older not covered by Medicare. No one is to be excluded on the basis of diagnosis. An exception is that federal funds cannot be used to support the care of those between ages 21 and 65 in a psychiatric institution or a psychiatric skilled nursing home. When Medicaid was enacted, most psychiatric patients were receiving care in state hospitals. Medicaid is a major funding source in many states for care of the young and the elderly in psychiatric hospitals. Twenty-three percent of the total population in nursing homes are considered to have a mental disorder (Taube, et al., 1990). Of the mentally ill nursing home resident population, 37 percent of those under age 65 and 27 percent of those aged 65 and older had Medicaid as their primary source of payment.

In contrast to Medicare, Medicaid has large outpatient care expenditures. The poor/near-poor with continuous Medicaid coverage had almost double the probability of use of ambulatory mental health care compared to the poor/near-poor not enrolled in Medicaid (Taube and Rupp, 1986). This in part reflects the impact of increased financial accessibility to needed mental health services and may be influenced by an associated demand for social services provided by organized mental health settings.

Furthermore, mentally ill Medicaid users differ from other users primarily in the greater intensity of their use of services and the greater number of heavy users (Dobson and Scharff-Corder, 1983). In 1980 less than 10 percent of the mentally ill Medicaid population generated more than one third of the treatment costs.

Medicaid has been a major source of revenue to providers of mental health services. Estimates indicate that about 15 percent of total Medicaid dollars were spent on mental illness in 1988. The bulk of costs included over $2 billion for skilled nursing facilities and intermediate care facilities, $2 billion for general hospital psychiatric care, and $1 billion for state psychiatric care (Koyanagi, 1988). Medicaid payment policy encourages the use of general hospital services over other settings for care and its rates come closer to covering costs for inpatient care than for ambulatory care. Consequently, some patients may be admitted to the hospital unnecessarily because appropriate outpatient services are unprofitable and unavailable.

Private Insurance

Private insurance to cover costs of hospitalization, but not physicians' fees, has its roots in Texas in 1929 at Baylor Hospital where a program was set up to insure teachers. During the Depression, private insurance through these nonprofit plans (called Blue Cross and tied to individual hospitals) grew quickly. Health insurance expanded further during World War II, when it was offered instead of wage increases during the wage/price freeze of the war. Private insurers included very liberal inpatient and outpatient psychiatric coverage, probably because most psychiatric treatment took place in public hospitals and little demand was expected. In the 1950s, however, with increased availability of services and a broadened concept of mental illness, private insurers noted large claims made for ambulatory psychiatric care. Consequently, private insurers imposed arbitrary limits on outpatient benefits for a population the insurers viewed as "healthy" people, and to a lesser extent limited hospital coverage. We will discuss private financing in two parts—retrospective payments made after a service has been given, and prospective payments in which fixed fees are paid to providers of care for a designated period whether or not services are used.

Retrospective Payment. It is difficult to assess the percentage of Americans who are covered by private insurance plans that pay for medical care after it has been given, because many people have more than one policy. The U.S. Bureau of Census estimated that 82 percent of the civilian population was covered by private health insurance in 1983.

In the most comprehensive overview to date of private indemnity insurance programs, Brady, et al. (1986) found that 99 percent of twenty million Bureau of Labor Statistics (BLS) survey participants working in medium and large firms received insurance coverage for inpatient psychiatric care, but fewer than half had coverage equal to that for other illnesses. Limitations on days of care have remained relatively constant, but an increasing number of employers cap psychiatric benefits; 15 percent did so in 1981 and 24 percent in 1984. Outpatient coverage for mental illness has probably deteriorated even though 97 percent of participants were covered in 1986 (Scheidemandel, 1989). Dollar limits on outpatient benefits per year and, to a lesser extent, per visit, continue to be the most commonly applied benefit limits, and many of these have not been increased in years, while treatment costs rise. Fifteen percent of participants had outpatient benefits limited to $25 or less per physician visit— less than one third of average charges in 1986. Only 10.7 percent of all participants were covered for day or night hospital treatment. Only 6 percent had coverage for psychiatric outpatient treatment equal to outpatient coverage for other illness; only 37 percent had coverage for psychiatric inpatient treatment on a par with that for other illness. Thus, much of the coverage in the current private sector fails to insure both the poor and the middle class against potential significant loss. Blue Cross and Blue Shield are estimated to insure roughly 40 percent of those with private insurance. Employers with hospital benefits insured by commercial carriers were more than twice as likely (63 percent vs. 30 percent) to have plans offering psychiatric benefits equal to medical benefits than those who were insured by Blue Cross and Blue Shield (Ridgely and Goldman, 1989).

Coverage for alcohol and drug abuse treatment increased considerably between 1983 and 1986; the proportion of BLS-surveyed employees with alcohol abuse coverage increased from 51 percent in 1983 to 70 percent in 1986, and the proportion covered for both alcohol and drug abuse rose from 40 percent in 1983 to 66 percent in 1986 (Scheidemandel, 1989).

Some states began mandating a certain amount of mental health insurance coverage in the early 1970s and by 1989, twenty-seven states and the District of Columbia had at least some mandated coverage, mostly for group policies (Scheidemandel, 1989). Large firms were increasingly self-insuring, which exempts them from state mandates. Those self-insurers surveyed by the BLS in 1989, however, were providing inpatient psychiatric coverage in general hospitals similar to or better than that offered by other insurance plans, but were less likely to offer coverage in specialty mental health facilities.

Private insurance carriers offered many options for mental health care. The number of days of care, number of visits, amount of deductibles, and coinsurance payments all vary. Insurers assume that much mental health care is discretionary and subject to overuse unless purchasers share the cost. We know that demand for mental health care is responsive to price; the higher the price to the consumer, the lower the utilization; price responsiveness decreases as income of patients increases, and is more responsive to price for mental health care than for general medical care (Wells, et al., 1986). However, this presumption that services are used unnecessarily does not separate discretionary from medically necessary use of psychiatric care forgone because of cost. The effect of insurance on access to care for individuals with addictions is poorly understood.

Private insurers, like public insurers, are eagerly searching for better methods of cost containment. There has been an increase in regulatory guidelines and activity in examining requests for reimbursement. Some insurers have now shifted to a prospective payment system of reimbursement.

Prospective Payment. The 1980s saw a large increase in enrollment in health maintenance organizations (HMO) from some 3 million in 1972 to over 30 million persons by 1988 (Shadle and Christianson, 1988). The HMO Act of 1973 provided government grants and subsidies to encourage what legislators viewed as a promising cost-cutting mechanism. In 1980 3 percent of all full-time workers in medium and large firms who were covered by employer-sponsored health insurance participated in HMOs, but by 1988 the number had grown to 19 percent (Levit, et al., 1990). HMOs are an organized system of providing comprehensive inpatient and outpatient health care. Members enroll by paying a fixed fee in advance of treatment for each person enrolled to cover all health services for a designated period of time. In this method of payment, called capitation, a provider receives a payment for each person served without regard to the amount or nature of the services provided. This shifts the burden of high utilization away from the insurer.

These arrangements emphasize the limiting of services and often manage the behavior of providers in supplying those services. To stay within budget, the HMO contracts with hospitals and sometimes with groups of independent physicians at a discount for its members and relies as well on utilization review of admissions and ongoing review of length and methods of treatment. Denial or rationing of care does occur. For example, in a majority of HMOs today there is a built-in screening mechanism that prevents the patient from receiving specialty mental health services until evaluation and referral by a primary care physician.

The HMO may also provide little or no psychiatric care (Levinson, 1987). This tactic has been adopted by HMOs in states that do not have mandated minimum inpatient mental health benefits. Restricting services poses special threats to patients who have major chronic disorders such as schizophrenia or Alzheimer's disease. Utilization review can be a threat to effective treatment if the reviewers are not well trained to evaluate care or are under corporate pressure to make restrictive decisions. Appeal mechanisms may be inadequate and reviews worry patients who fear loss of confidentiality (Borenstein, 1990).

There is little uniformity of services among the many different forms of HMOs, making it difficult for patients to evaluate knowledgeably the quality of benefits offered by the plan even if the amount of the benefits is specified. Although further comparisons should be made, our review shows that there appear to be more exclusions, a narrower range of service benefits, and less intensive, short-term care by mental health providers in HMOs than in non-HMO insurance programs (Dorwart and Epstein, 1992).

While HMO managers are under pressure to offer fewer expensive services than would an unmanaged insurance plan, they must also respond to demand for services from their enrollees who pay a fixed price. Thus, controlling demand is a critical factor in meeting budget, leading managers to target memberships to groups perceived to have low utilization rates.

Despite these problems, patients with psychiatric difficulties may benefit from being seen in HMOs. The multidisciplinary practice and the varied modes of therapy associated with HMOs, especially in group or staff models, mean that a patient's disorder may receive team evaluation and consultation, and the most appropriate treatments are likely to be more convenient and accessible than in a solo practitioner setting. The HMO may also be able to provide care more cost-effectively through the use of non-physician services or low-cost treatment such as group therapy. Both approaches were adopted by the Group Health Cooperative studied by health economist at the Rand Corporation research study group (Wells, et al., 1986). Costs may also be affected by increased productivity of clinical staff; a recent study showed 80 percent of HMO staff time spent in direct care (Shadle and Christianson, 1988).

NEW AND FUTURE DEVELOPMENTS

Managed Care and Utilization Review

The desire by government, private insurers, and employers to control the rising costs of medical care has made "managed care" a byword for cost containment rather than a description of a program that—in its "purist" definition—determines the most appropriate and efficient treatment for the patient in question (Dorwart, 1990). Costs for psychiatric and substance abuse services are said to be growing more rapidly than are those for other types of medical care (Frank, et al., 1991), making these services vulnerable to the calls for increased managed care (Pepper Commission, 1990). Even advocates for such care sound cautionary notes, however, advising the necessity of choosing the right delivery model, appropriate providers, careful financial incentives, and proper oversight (Patterson, 1990).

Utilization review is becoming increasingly important for psychiatric care in all settings. Retrospective review occurs in which reimbursement may be denied for services deemed unnecessary, and providers and reviewers often must discuss patient care during treatment (concurrent review). These review mechanisms tend to emphasize the most efficient and "proven" treatments, not always the ones psychiatrists would choose to address the special needs of particular patients. Professional uncertainty and discretionary behavior occur throughout medical practice, but professional judgment is especially valued and consensus difficult to achieve in psychiatry, as Tischler explains (Tischler, 1990). Utilization review is "a direct effort to regulate and control physicians by modifying their decisions," says Sharfstein (Sharfstein, 1990), accounting for the resentment of it felt by psychiatrists. While he sees value in coordinating specialized treatment for difficult patients to insure quality care at the lowest cost, he claims that the majority of utilization management is geared toward "cost containment pure and simple." Reviewers may require details about the patient's condition to prove need of treatment that conflict with confidentiality, as Morreim and Tischler discuss (Morreim, 1990; Tischler, 1990). Managed care and utilization review, with their emphasis on insuring quality of care and keeping costs down, are unlikely to disappear from the psychiatric care scene even though their effectiveness in either sphere is far from proven. Better evaluation of its effects must be carried out so that psychiatrists can accommodate its rational aspects and resist those that are harmful.

Managed care is most often delivered through HMOs, thus helping to change the concept of the HMO from its earlier focus on preventive health care to its current one on limiting costs by setting reimbursement rates for a predetermined set of services. Subscribers pay a fixed fee in advance for a designated period of time, shifting the burden of high utilization, when it occurs, away from the insurer and to the provider. These arrangements thus tend to limit services and often regulate the behavior of the doctors or other health care providers who must stay within budget. Regulation is carried out through screening of admissions and ongoing review of length and type of treatment. When reviewers are not well trained to evaluate psychiatric care, or are pressured by business considerations, inappropriate short-term admissions may occur; appeal mechanisms are often inadequate, and reviews often risk confidentiality (Borenstein, 1990). In states that do not have mandated minimum inpatient mental health benefits, the HMO may provide little or no psychiatric care (Levinson, 1987). The incentive for providers under these so-called prospective reimbursement plans is to treat lower cost (less ill) patients; serious mental illness is unlikely to be well served under present arrangements (Ridgely, et al., 1990).

Capitation Plans

The era of fiscal constraints on health care services is likely to persist into the 1990s. Advocates of better mental health care are experimenting with various capitation plans that they hope will coordinate care among the various levels of government and social service agencies at the same time that mental health dollars are spent more effectively. Under capitation, providers of care are paid a fixed amount in advance for each client served during the year regardless of the amount of care needed. The proposed capitation plans have included mainstreaming the mentally ill into general HMOs, developing HMOs specifically for the mentally ill, designating preferred providers who provide care for a prepaid fee, and federal and state planning that allows a capitation approach to the care of the severely mentally ill—dollars follow the patients to provide a support system in the community (Talbott and Sharfstein, 1986). Capitation plans can offer a financial and organizational framework that substantially aids case managers in performing their function. Unfortunately, in practice, capitation has been difficult to establish and to manage: as in more traditional HMOs, prepayment may provide incentives for inadequate care; if the risk pool is not large enough and prepayments have been set too low, the plans will have trouble meeting costs. The capitation experiment carried out in Rochester, New York, however, offers a promising example of the flexible control of services possible in a well designed and adequately financed plan (Babigian and Marshall, 1989). Other demonstration projects based on capitation may also show they can deliver improved mental health services cost effectively, but have not been in effect long enough for evaluation (Hadley, et al., 1989).

Diagnosis-Related Groups and Psychiatry

The American Psychiatric Association (APA) studies have demonstrated that the diagnosis-related group (DRG) approach to cost saving instituted by Medicare in the 1980s to determine in advance the allowed cost of a patient's illness was not, in 1991, well-defined enough to be implemented for the majority of psychiatric patients (Cromwell, et al., 1991). Research to find a hospital payment system that will be an alternative to cost-based reimbursement will continue. It is also predicted that setting psychiatrists' fees will be seen as another method of cost saving. It is expected that the government study to determine a relative value scale for physicians' services will affect psychiatrists' fees.

Resource-Based Relative Value Scale (RBRVS)

Health care payment reform in the 1990s seems likely to center on the way in which individual physicians are reimbursed for services. The federal Health Care Financing Administration (HCFA) is taking the lead in stimulating this reform in collaboration with researchers at the Harvard School of Public Health. Under the direction of health economist Hsiao (1988), a new methodology for financing physician services was developed, called the resource-based relative value scale (Dorwart and Chartock, 1988). Although this system of payment reflects the basic structure of a fee-for-service or market-based approach, there are also significant differences. The RBRVS attempts to adjust the amount of payment for physician services according to the actual labor input or "work" involved in providing a particular service. The aim is to readjust compensation to reward primary care and evaluation of patients more and to reward performance of procedures less. The estimates of these resource inputs are based on extensive survey research conducted by the Hsiao team for each of twenty-three medical specialties, including psychiatry. Results of these studies are being implemented according to guidelines in the 1989 Federal Physician Payment Reform Act. This approach to changing compensation patterns provides an important model for understanding future directions in physician payment, not only under Medicare but throughout the health care system. Other insurers have typically followed Medicare's lead.

In the course of the development of an RBRVS for psychiatry, it became apparent that the existing specification of psychiatric services most widely used for reimbursement purposes (the AMA's *Current Procedural Terminology*, 4th Ed. codes) were inadequate to describe the range and diversity and subtlety of services provided by psychiatrists. The most glaring example of this deficiency was the codes used for psychotherapy, in which a 50-minute individual medical-psychotherapy service was used generically for all office visits of 50-minutes duration and accounted for nearly 50 percent of all outpatient mental health services provided by psychiatrists under Medicare. With the development of the RBRVS, it may be possible to segment such broad categories of services into a more differentiated system of classification based on difficulty of the services provided. Researchers at the Physician Payment Review Commission, the American Medical Association, and the American Psychiatric Association are working collaboratively to develop other approaches to improving financing mechanisms. An intriguing but unanswered question is whether changes in the coding system will lead to changes in practice for services provided by psychiatrists and other physicians. The impact of the RBRVS reform on the access to care and the volume and types of care provided will be an important area for research.

Children and Mental Illness

The number of children with chronic illnesses has more than doubled since the 1960s, according to a number of researchers, who attribute it to various causes, including advances in neonatal care that allow survival at a cost. Estimates are that 11 percent of U.S. children need mental health treatment (Saxe, et al., 1988) and in addition, chronic physical illnesses bring with them the need for mental health counseling. Insurance benefits provided by employers for mental health care of workers' dependents were shown in a recent survey to be significantly more restrictive than those for other health benefits (Fox and Newacheck, 1990). Half the employers placed limits on the number of visits and one-third specified coverage with certain dollar limits.

Hospitalization rates of children with mental illness have increased in the 1980s, with hospital care shifting from the public sector to the private. As with adults, the majority of psychiatric inpatient episodes for children in the United States occur in short-term general hospitals (Kiesler, et al., 1989). But children, according to Kiesler, despite more complex psychiatric diagnoses, are more likely than adults to be treated in scatter beds where they may not be seen by psychiatrists rather than in specialty psychiatric units; they stay in hospitals longer than adults, and are substantially more likely to pay for care with commercial insurance. Since estimates are that only a small fraction of children in need receive mental health treatment, Kiesler concludes that inpatient treatment is tilted toward middle-class children.

Provision of more community-based services for children who do not need intensive treatment has long been called for by presidential commissions and national panels, but has not taken place—largely because payment for mental health treatment has come increasingly from health insurance, which typically pays for some hospitalization but is restrictive in providing outpatient or non-medical residential treatment. Kiesler estimates that over $1 billion of the $1.5 billion paid for inpatient care of children in 1989 came from commercial insurers and might well not represent the most cost effective expenditure these companies could have made.

The hope that HMOs might be a source of more easily accessed and better coordinated health care for children who need mental health services is not borne out by several recent studies (Valdez, et al., 1989; Horwitz and Stein, 1990). The Horwitz and Stein survey of Connecticut insurers found that both HMOs and conventional insurers used case managers to control expenses rather than to coordinate services; both restricted mental health services for children, and both predicted greater restrictions in the future. The findings were especially disturbing because Connecticut mandates generous minimum standards for insurance compared to other states, and takes regulation seriously.

Financing of Substance Abuse Treatment

Changes in the way substance abuse treatment is organized and financed have been proposed in a 1990 study by the Institute of Medicine (Gerstein and Harwood, 1990). The National Institute on Drug Abuse (NIDA) funded this evaluation of public and private funding for treating abusers of illicit drugs. The findings indicate that public programs have paid for themselves by reducing crime and deserve additional funding to reduce waiting lists for methadone maintenance treatment and other treatment programs, especially those for criminals and for pregnant addicts. The study committee argued that federal contributions for public treatment programs have been inadequate and should be increased substantially. They urged that the federal government require state Medicaid programs to include drug abuse treatment as a standard benefit. Less favorable were the findings about private inpatient treatment programs, especially those based in hospitals.

The committee's report found little evidence that the results of inpatient treatment in private hospitals merited the added expense over out-of-hospital residential treatment or outpatient sessions. Better evaluation studies of treatment modalities are needed to see if inpatient care for drug abuse is justified under particular circumstances. The study drew on a 1987 NIDA survey that found the public tier of the drug treatment system treating three times as many people as the private tier at half the cost per episode. Committee members cautioned that the public facilities have been operating at greatly reduced federal contributions since 1975 and that although their case load has not diminished, their facilities, services, and personnel are all less than adequate to the task of delivering quality service.

Comorbidity with substance abuse. The inability of the seriously mentally ill to negotiate the multiple organizations that make up the mental health system has been discussed many times, recently explained well by Bloche and Cournos (Bloche and Cournos, 1990). The problem is compounded when the patient's mental illness is complicated by substance abuse—a common occurrence, with 53 percent of those in the NIMH's ECA study who abused drugs found to be also suffering from a mental disorder (Regier, et al., 1990). The difficulties faced by these patients in adapting to the way mental health services are organized by category is delineated well by Ridgely and co-authors, who also point out the likelihood of exclusion of poor, complicated patients from the growing number of private hospitals. Third-party funding, both public and private, is often lacking or severely restricted; both the Veterans Administration and the Social Security Administration limit benefits for those disabled by alcohol and drug abuse. The authors' suggestions for solving the difficulties of patients with comorbidities hinge on cooperative agreements among agencies and they cite some examples. Perhaps a policy suggestion more likely to be acted on is their support of contracting with private specialty providers for services for this group—a less expensive approach, they claim, than expecting public agencies to set up special services for them. Other authors agree that contracting represents a means by which public sector patients may gain access to private providers (Fisher, et al., 1991).

Drug abuse. Over the past decade there has been increasing public attention in the United States to the dangers of substance abuse. More than 500,000 Americans are admitted each year to community hospitals with a primary diagnosis of physical illness and a secondary diagnosis that involved drug abuse problems (Rice and Kelman, 1989). Between 1980 and 1986 the number of general hospitals with chemical dependency units more than doubled. Insurance-based financing has focused on short-term treatment for a problem that may be lifelong, resulting in recycling of patients, as evidenced by the Veterans Administration experience (Rosenheck, et al., 1990).

SUMMARY

It is likely that in the future both private and public mental health care will be driven by cost containment considerations. In the private sector, employers and insurers are increasingly unwilling to expand benefits for any kind of health care; mental health benefits have traditionally lagged behind those available for other illness and there seems little prospect that this will change. The 1989 Health Insurance Association of America (HIAA) survey that sampled 2,600 firms found a slight decline from the previous year in coverage of mental health benefits. Insurers and the employers who pay the bulk of health insurance charges are urging subscribers to choose plans perceived to be less costly, such as health maintenance plans, by offering incentives over fee-for-service choices. Arbitrary limits on psychiatric outpatient visits are the rule because insurers fear overuse; instead, the necessity of visits could be evaluated and copayments adjusted accordingly. Some attempt at this has been shown by Medicare's willingness to pay on a par with medical treatment for visits that involve adjustment of psychiatric medications.

Public mental health services are provided by diverse programs that have multiplied over the years, funded through federal, state, and local entities, and are largely uncoordinated. The federal share of funding for public services, including the disability income programs, made up some 40 percent of the total in 1990 (Torrey, et al., 1990). Although state mental health authorities are struggling to provide adequate services under declining national and state economies, their attempts at coordinating the various programs are unlikely to be successful unless the funding regulations of the federal government—especially for Medicaid—are brought into compliance with current theories of treatment. The integration of public and private systems of care and of divergent financing streams must be a priority of future mental health policy.

PART II _____

OWNERSHIP AND ACCESS TO CARE: A NATIONAL PERSPECTIVE

CHAPTER 4 _____

The Privatization Era

Privatization is a term that has been applied both to the growing number of private nonprofit and for-profit facilities carrying out mental health care and the increasing purchase by public authorities of services from private agencies. Purchase of services has occurred in areas of social services other than mental health where government agencies have traditionally been the providers.

Examples of privatization in government include: port authorities and air traffic control, the postal service, AMTRAK rail service, housing and education programs, and various health and social service programs. Privatization has been defined as the use of private means to further public ends (Donahue, 1989). In privatizing services, market-oriented economic principles are employed in an effort to make government more cost effective in pursuit of its goals. One of the largest of the government's social programs, costing about $100 billion annually, is Medicare, the administration of which embodies many of the major features of privatization, such as: contracting with private providers for goods and services;

We acknowledge with gratitude the substantial contributions to this chapter and the next two made by our long-time colleague, Mark Schlesinger, Ph.D., now an Associate Professor at the Yale University School of Medicine. He was responsible for much of the design and analysis of the National Mental Health Facilities study (see Chapter 5), and we have drawn upon published papers on hospital ownership and privatization written with him in preparing these chapters.

providing vouchers in the form of insurance benefits to individuals who can then choose among competing providers of services; and relying on the private sector to ensure efficiency, innovativeness, and consumer satisfaction.

Recently, there has been increasing interest in the provision of public mental health services under private auspice: in private specialty hospitals, in general hospitals, and in mental health centers and clinics. Paradoxically, proponents and opponents of privatization argue that privatization will either positively, or negatively, affect access to care, costs of care, quality of care, and accountability for the delivery of care. It is undisputed, however, that the increasing reliance on private payment or insurance sources of revenue puts pressure on all types of psychiatric hospitals. Public hospitals are forced to accept a large proportion of poor, seriously mentally ill patients who are difficult to treat and expensive to care for because both private profit-making and nonprofit providers are forced to avoid admitting those who are uninsured or so costly to treat that their insurance benefits may run out.

Public insurers (Medicaid and Medicare) and private insurance companies both pressure hospitals to "manage" well and to be more "business-like" in holding costs down. Medicaid, a major payer for care of the indigent mentally ill, is the victim of tight federal and state budgets and increasingly makes conflicting demands for efficiency and cost containment from mental health authorities (Taube, et al., 1990). Similarly, cost considerations limit the number who receive care paid for by Medicare for disability from mental illness (Lave and Goldman, 1990). Although there are advantages to increasing efficiency, emphasis on reducing costs tends to create barriers both to access to and quality of care for the poor, the elderly, and the seriously mental ill. Several recent studies have also emphasized how difficult it is to make cost evaluations for mental health services in the United States and in England (Feis, et al., 1990; Scallett, 1990; Knapp and Beecham, 1990). Morreim outlines well the dilemma faced in psychiatry by the economic pressures to raise revenues and to fill hospital beds occurring at the same time that controls and incentives to contain costs are being imposed by insurers (Morreim, 1990). We will consider the implications of privatization in health care generally and more specifically its impact on mental health services.

THE EVOLUTION OF PRIVATIZATION

The privatization trend affecting the psychiatric hospital industry has been an outgrowth of broader changes in the American health care system.

Among these has been a growing concern about the financial well-being of community hospitals. Between 1980 and 1985, occupancy rates in community hospitals fell from 75.6 precent to 64.8 percent and these rates are continuing to decline. Prospective hospital payment using diagnosis-related groups (DRGs) was introduced nationwide under Medicare in 1983, and many states adopted similar systems for their Medicaid programs. Most observers anticipated that these payment restrictions would result in declining income for hospitals delivering general health care. By comparison, psychiatric services appeared to many to be a significantly more profitable market. Most of the increase in general hospital psychiatric units nationally has taken the form of units exempt from current Medicare prospective payment regulations and those in which sagging occupancy rates were driving conversion of medical beds to psychiatric beds.

This shift from general to mental health care has been stimulated by the growth of multifacility health care systems. Many of these systems, and virtually all of the investor-owned variety, were first incorporated in the late 1960s. They grew most rapidly throughout the 1970s. By the mid-1980s, however, the growth of all systems among community general hospitals had begun to slow, particularly among the investor-owned systems, which had acquired all the readily available general hospitals.

The limited potential for expansion of general hospitals encouraged systems to shift their purchasing power into the market for psychiatric services. Inpatient mental health care promised higher occupancy rates than in general acute care hospitals, less costly operations, less regulation under prospective payment mechanisms, and the ability to transfer difficult and expensive patients to public facilities. By the mid-1980s, about half of the psychiatric specialty hospitals in this country were operated by systems that included both psychiatric and general hospitals. A number of the psychiatric inpatient units in general hospitals were also operated by multifacility corporations.

Other factors fostering the shift of mental health care services from public to private settings resulted from explicit decisions made by public officials, usually at the state level. Deinstitutionalization resulted in increased demand for psychiatric services in local community hospitals and encouraged private vendors to provide community support services like crisis intervention, aftercare, and residential treatment. Between 1980 and 1985, when the overall demand for mental health care facilities was on the rise, the number of state and local beds designated for long-term psychiatric care fell by 29 percent; beds designated for short-term care declined by 15 percent.

Much of the expansion of privately-owned facilities was the explicit intent of state policymakers, who often judged private providers to have higher quality and lower costs than their government-operated counterparts. State contracts often paid the costs of services complementary to inpatient treatment—e.g., aftercare or emergency services—that may either increase a hospital's caseload or decrease the ancillary costs associated with operating a psychiatric facility. Either makes private psychiatric hospitals more financially viable.

The expansion of private mental health has been promoted, too, as states have loosened or eliminated their certificate-of-need requirements for new hospital construction. Over half the new hospitals being built by one of the nation's largest psychiatric hospital systems were located in states that had dropped certificate-of-need laws in the 1980s.

Finally, privatization has increased because demand for psychiatric treatment has grown more socially acceptable. While mental illness still carries some stigma, this has diminished over past decades, as the general public became more knowledgeable about mental illness and adopted the concept that health, including mental health, care is a universal right or entitlement. As public acceptance of psychiatric care increased, so did the willingness to seek services for "new" diseases like eating, panic, stress, or addictive disorders. The value placed on mental health has led to a wish for access to psychiatric and psychological services to obtain help in coping with interpersonal or societal stresses, as well as with major psychiatric or substance abuse disorders.

The increased acceptance of treatment as a marketable commodity has helped reduce the social stigma of mental illness. As medical and mental health care have become more commercialized, there has been an increased willingness among providers to actively market their services. This emphasis on marketing—generally defined as the art and science of creating a demand for goods and services—further induces demand for these services.

The Effect of Changes in the Financing of Health Care

Patients in the U.S. health care system have long relied on the kindness of strangers. Before the introduction of health insurance in the 1930s, much of the medical care in this country was financed through philanthropy or grants from local government. As health insurance became more common, private providers used the revenues produced by insured patients to cover the costs of those without coverage. But recent competitive pressures have, over time, begun to change the practices of insurers, employers, and health care providers. This has left each less willing to bear the medical costs of the poor and uninsured. As a result, gaps have emerged in the private "safety net" for health care, gaps that increasingly threaten the health and well-being of disadvantaged Americans and that raise new questions about the appropriate roles of public and private sectors in financing and delivering health services.

American medicine is largely financed and delivered through the private sector. Historically, private employers, insurers, and medical practitioners have contributed an important public service by providing health care for those unable to pay on their own. This is a vital role that continues; thirty-five million Americans are uninsured and obtain what health care they receive through charity, typically in an emergency room setting. This includes a disproportionate number of children (11.7 million uninsured) and minorities (6.5 million uninsured). An equal number have insurance so limited that they face potentially catastrophic medical costs if they become seriously ill and if collection procedures are pursued.

Without adequate health insurance, the costs of medical care can be daunting. But while the uninsured use less health care, historically they have been able to obtain needed services. In a 1982 survey, only 6 percent of the uninsured who had a medical emergency reported that they had problems obtaining care; less than 4 percent of the uninsured indicated that they had been refused medical care for financial reasons. This treatment, though, entailed significant societal costs—providers incur between $15 and $20 billion annually in uncompensated expenses.

But this traditional role for the private sector may be disappearing. The behavior of insurers, employers, and practitioners has become increasingly "privatized," that is, focused on their own economic well-being rather than their broader societal role to provide health care for the poor. This narrowing of vision has occurred as private entities faced competitive pressures that forced them to become more cognizant of the "bottom line."

Increased competition and more "business like" approaches to administration in the health care system can have some important benefits, motivating providers to satisfy the preferences of those purchasing care. But they also have created significant new barriers to health care for the poor. Between 1982 and 1986, for example, the number of Americans who had not seen a physician at all in the previous year rose from forty-two million to eighty million. Getting to a medical practitioner was only half the battle—increasingly, providers have been turning away patients who were unable to pay for care. Reports from a number of cities indicate that the number of patients discharged from private hospitals for purely economic reasons more than tripled during the early 1980s.

These financial barriers have their greatest effects on those most vulnerable to the problems created by inadequate medical care. A 1987 survey of low-income women with inadequate prenatal care found that 25 percent had not sought care earlier due to financial factors, 10 percent hadn't delivered the baby at the hospital of their choice because it required a preadmission financial deposit, and 9 percent had been unable to find a physician who was willing to treat them. Between 1982 and 1986, the number of children without a regular source of medical care doubled. Racial differentials in access to care, which had been steadily narrowing since the mid-1960s, began to reemerge. During this same time period, the difference in the number of physician visits for whites in fair and poor health, compared to blacks with equal health status, grew by more than 25 percent.

Privatization and Public Policy. These statistics make clear that the informal norms and practices upon which the poor and uninsured, many of whom have incomes barely above welfare levels, have so long relied to pay for medical care are rapidly eroding in the face of competitive pressures within American medicine. Two strategies can be pursued to repair the tattered private safety net: regulation and the substitution of public programs for private actions.

The regulatory approach has taken two directions. A number of states have prohibited medical providers from turning away patients based on economic criteria, requiring that they be treated at least until their medical conditions are stabilized. Hawaii requires that employers offer health insurance as a benefit for their workers. Senator Edward Kennedy of Massachusetts and others have introduced congressional legislation that would establish similar requirements nationwide.

Undoubtedly the regulatory approach could improve access for some patients. But it also has some very real limitations. One cannot force providers to offer additional unprofitable care when competition has eroded their financial surplus. And it is often the providers who have traditionally offered the most uncompensated care who are now in the worst financial position. There are few advantages to mandated insurance benefits if requiring employers to add 5 to 10 percent to their labor costs drives them out of business or forces them to hire fewer workers. When Massachusetts considered regulating employers, it was found that almost half of the currently uninsured population would be excluded from mandated insurance plans because they were in households where the primary wage-earner was either unemployed, a part-time worker, or worked for a small business that could not afford the costs of health insurance. Those excluded would be disproportionately from the lowest income levels.

These considerations lead to the conclusion that some new public programs for financing health care are inevitable. Just as the privatization of health insurance represented by experience rating in the 1950s led to Medicare for the elderly, so too the ongoing privatization of financing and delivery systems creates the need for new public programs for the uninsured. Although interest in national health insurance, dormant in this country since the mid-1970s, has been reawakened in the 1990s, the most promising short-term avenue seems to lie in recent experiments with reforming Medicaid eligibility. Several states have established pilot programs under which Medicaid is converted from a welfare-based program to one through which insurance can be purchased by anyone, with premiums that are adjusted for family income. This sort of Medicaid conversion could successfully fill a major gap in existing insurance arrangements, making insurance affordable to the working poor. It would allow those now on welfare to take jobs without losing Medicaid insurance coverage. It would also make proposals for mandated employer benefits more practical. Small employers with low-wage workers could buy Medicaid coverage for their workers; by so doing, government would share the costs of providing insurance.

Privatization and Psychiatric Hospital Care

A marked shift toward care of the mentally ill in private facilities rather than publicly owned hospitals has occurred in the United States since the 1970s. Whereas twenty years ago, 95 percent of the much larger number of psychiatric beds were government operated, fewer that 50 percent of the beds are government owned today. The number of private psychiatric hospitals has multiplied from 184 in 1979 to an estimate of more than 450 in 1990 (Dorwart, et al., 1991). Proprietary (for-profit) hospitals, largely specialty facilities, numbered 88 in 1979 but some 350 by 1988. Most are operated by investor-owned systems and are concentrated in southern and western states. Our National Mental Health Facilities study (see Chapter 5) found for-profit hospitals less likely than others to provide potentially unprofitable services, i.e., those desirable for patients with chronic disorders but unlikely to be paid for fully. Private hospitals treated a lower proportion of patients with schizophrenia and a higher proportion with depression than did public hospitals, reflecting the private hospitals' preference for patients who can be treated in relatively short periods. Specialty, for-profit hospitals seemed to be filling a previous gap in treating children and adolescents, although questions arise about excessive hospitalization where outpatient treatment might suffice (Weithorn, 1988).

Other trends evident from the National Mental Health Facilities study are the increasing share of costs paid in all settings by government insurance (Medicare and Medicaid), a general improvement in quality of care measured by the number of patients-to-professional staffs in all hospitals, and the increasing medicalization of psychiatry, especially in general hospitals.

Short-term general hospitals emerged as the most likely place for hospitalization for mental illness in the mid-1980s (Wallen, 1986). The sources of funds for mental health service have to a large extent determined where care is given, with private insurance coverage driving the growth in private psychiatric hospitals and Medicaid rules that preclude payment for adults in public hospitals spurring the growth in general hospital care for the mentally ill. General hospitals can maximize their resources by using excess bed capacity for patients with psychiatric illness. These hospitals, laboring under prospective payment rules instituted by Medicare in 1982, also may find that psychiatric patients are more profitable than general medical/surgical patients when they are treated in scatter beds rather than in an organized psychiatric unit, although it may only be possible to treat patients who are not very ill in scatter beds (Freiman, 1990). Frank and Kamlet concluded that care in the specialty hospital is from three to twenty times more expensive than that provided in the general hospital, but are not convinced that caring for a needier population explains the difference (Frank and Kamlet, 1990). They suggest that studies that might show better outcomes to justify the expense remain to be done.

The proportion of psychiatric patients in general hospitals with a diagnosis of severe mental illness has been shown to have increased substantially from 1970 to 1980, burdening general hospitals with patients formerly treated in state institutions (Salit and Marcos, 1991). Olfson, however, claims that severity of mental illness among general hospital patients has remained stable between 1980 and 1986; he attributes an apparent increase to changes in the American Psychiatric Association's *Diagnostic and Statistical Manual of Mental Disorders*, 3rd Ed. classifications (Olfson, 1991).

IMPLICATIONS OF PRIVATIZATION AND RELATED TRENDS

Privatization is the 1980s' socioeconomic megatrend affecting health care and psychiatry. Megatrends result from a combination of socioeconomic, scientific, or political developments in society that bring about a major shift in the nature of a field. The megatrend synthesizes what might otherwise appear only as disparate developments. "Deinstitutionalization" is an example of such a megatrend in mental health services and public policy in the 1970s.

In their book *Megatrends 2000*, Naisbitt and Aburdene (1990) identify "privatization of welfare services" as one of the ten new directions of change in society in the 1990s, but as we have shown, this trend was already evident for psychiatric hospital services in the 1980s. The number of private, free-standing, psychiatric specialty hospitals (many of them for-profit businesses) tripled to more than 450. The number of psychiatric units in private, nonprofit, community general hospitals doubled to more than 1,500. At the same time, many states were "privatizing" their state mental health services by purchasing care under contract from private providers. Many other factors also contributed to this growth of the private mental health care sector.

Privatization in health care grew rapidly in the 1980s, fostered by federal and state social and health care policies promoting competition, deregulation, and cost containment. Changes in the delivery of psychiatric services are resulting from a shifting emphasis from the public (non-market) to the private (market) sectors. Our National Mental Health study examines the implications of a more than threefold increase in the number of private, free-standing psychiatric hospitals since 1955.

Purchase of services for public-care patients by government via contracts with private providers (degovernmentalization) is also a rapidly growing trend in many states, as is the growth of multihospital-system companies and the increasing involvement of physicians as investors in, and owners of, proprietary mental health care facilities (Eisenberg, 1984). Accompanying the marked expansion of new private and proprietary facilities are other changes, such as substitution of private for public, and outpatient for inpatient, capacities, as well as joint ventures between providers, with overlapping of services between the two sectors.

Besides privatization, there have been several other "megatrends" affecting the development of mental health services in the United States in the 1980s. A second trend is specialization and diversification, especially in the growth of organized settings for providing care from roughly 3,000 in 1970 to nearly twice that many today (NIMH, 1990a); for example, clinics, day-treatment programs, HMOs and group practices have grown rapidly during the past decade. In addition to specialized treatment programs—for children, drug abusers, elderly, eating-disorder patients and so forth—there has also been a growth in specialty treatments provided by individual practitioners. At the same time, in community mental health centers, a comprehensive agency now offers a wide range of specialty services (see also Chapter 7). A study by Woy, et al. (1981) found that after federal funding was phased out, many CMHCs moved toward self-sufficiency by evolving into privately funded agencies and by expanding the range of services offered. A third trend has been medicalization, as illustrated by the increasing emphasis on hospital treatments and greater reliance on general hospital units for providing services. Within these units, there is a tendency toward the use of modern neuropsychiatric/diagnostic evaluation involving new technologies, treatments based on somatic therapies and services based on an acute-care or medical model. A fourth trend, grounded in prevailing ideas about health policy and economics, is increasing competition in the medical marketplace. Competition is seen by many policymakers and administrators as a way to control costs, foster efficiency, improve quality, and increase access. In particular, a variety of administrative practices and financing mechanisms are being used in an attempt to increase competition, such as purchases of service contracting, utilization reviews, resource-based relative value scales, and creation of "public-private partnerships." One of the hopes for increasing competition is that it will foster more innovative approaches to the financing and organization of care. A fifth trend which has become apparent over the past decade is an increasing emphasis on managed care both in hospitals and among private providers, including the treatment of individuals with major mental illnesses.

Impact on Psychiatrists

What is the impact of these trends on psychiatric services for psychiatrists in practice? Individual psychiatrists are faced with such familiar concerns as retaining professional autonomy, coping with changes in the nature of clinical practice and working conditions, and resisting financial incentives that adversely influence practice patterns.

For physicians, professional autonomy has been a cornerstone of medical practice. Paul Starr, in analyzing the medical profession, has described how individual autonomy has eroded as medical advances brought with them growth of health care as an industry (Starr, 1982). One example is the change in decision making in hospitals; non-physician administrators interpreting cost cutting measures by insurers now often question physicians' orders for patient care. The general trend toward increased management of practice in organized medicine is another dimension of change. This increased organizational management characterizes many settings, including HMOs, Veterans' hospitals, state and county hospitals, and community hospitals and mental health centers. The degree of influence of corporate organizations on physician practices varies considerably, however, with some organizations allowing more autonomy than others.

In the early 1980s, according to data from the APA, more than half of active psychiatrists reported their primary work setting to be private practice and one-third of the others reported their secondary work setting as private practice. In addition, a recent survey suggested that nearly half of psychiatrists said they had no significant hospital affiliations for treating patients, confirming the importance of independent private practice in psychiatry. As recently as 1982, fewer than 4 percent of psychiatrists reported their primary work setting to be a private psychiatric hospital, a general hospital, or an HMO. But given the rate of change in health care and what we know of the growth of private hospitals, HMOs, and general hospital units, we can confidently predict that in the 1990s these patterns of practice settings also will change dramatically. What is less clear but critically important is how the change of setting and auspices will affect the professional autonomy of psychiatrists.

Financial Incentives and Arrangements. Numerous studies have documented that the annual income of psychiatrists makes them among the lowest-paid physicians. Psychiatrists' earnings in the private sector, however, have been higher than salaries in public facilities or universities. Since there is competition for psychiatric services, one of the effects of the growth of private sector mental health care logically should be an increase in average salaries of psychiatrists. Competition from private hospitals may force states and universities to reassess their salary scales in order to keep their personnel. Reimbursement rates for psychiatrists cannot be predicted confidently, however, because there is increasing pressure from government, employers, and insurers to scrutinize all physician reimbursement in the general effort to reduce medical costs.

Physicians' services account for more than 20 percent of national expenditures for health services and supplies. In practice, many physicians have multiple sources of income and a variety of complicated arrangements combining fee-for-service and salaried compensation, which usually rises in line with the physician's experience. Most non-salaried psychiatrists customarily receive incomes from a combination of patient fees (40 percent), commercial insurance (25 percent), Blue Cross-Blue Shield (20 percent) and government insurance programs (10–15 percent). On average, psychiatrists receive a smaller proportion of income from hospital-based services than do other physicians. It has long been argued that changes in economic incentives for physicians influence both physician practice patterns and access to care by patients.

Increasingly, physician compensation in hospitals is based not simply on fee-for-service or a salary, but on a salary plus incentives. Physicians may be offered a percent of gross or net departmental or hospital billings or a fixed percentage of charges as an incentive to increase overall earnings. Corporate hospital practices are likely to involve variations on salaried forms of compensation such as profit-sharing, contingency fees, and non-monetary benefits. A survey by the American Medical Association found that such arrangements occurred in 28 percent of proprietary hospitals and in 20 percent of system-affiliated hospitals.

Currently, driven by cost-containment pressures, hospitals and insurers have proposed altering fee-for-service models by paying physicians fixed amounts based on diagnosis-related groups, capitation formulas, or relative value scales (Dorwart and Chartock, 1988). Physicians are also being encouraged to undertake joint ventures or to go "at risk" with the hospital in group practice contracts with HMOs or large self-insured employers. These arrangements have potential pitfalls for psychiatrists who often find themselves adrift in what they perceive to be uncharted waters.

Patterns of Practice. Patterns of practice and treatment of patients are changing rapidly. These changes are due not only to privatization but also to many forces encouraging change in similar directions. For example, except for those engaged only in evaluation assessment and consultation, active psychiatrists reported that they spend 75 percent of their treatment hours providing some form of psychotherapy (including psychoanalysis). Significantly, nearly half (45 percent) of these treatment hours serve patients who are taking medications. In organized settings psychiatrists are encouraged to emphasize medical management of patients over more time-consuming psychotherapy. Interestingly, the typical psychiatrist, regardless of affiliation with a public or private facility, spends twenty-five hours per week providing direct patient care. What is less well documented is how the nature of patient care differs from one setting to another in terms of the diagnoses of patients seen, treatment modalities used, nonpatient-care time allocated, and pressures on practice patterns exerted.

Increasingly, patient-care activities are subjected both to peer review and utilization review by independent outside agents. Insurance company requirements dictate not only prior approval for admission but also lengths of stay, appropriate procedures and tests, and comparison of practices to statistical norms in the hospital or the region. These activities are by no means new, but they are increasing in use both in private and public hospitals. Often, financial incentives (e.g., contracts or risk pools) or insurer regulations (e.g., pre-admission screening, concurrent review) are designed to encourage use of particular hospitals, specific treatments, or even to discourage the treatment of some common disorders. The psychiatrist is often caught in the middle, trying ethically to resolve conflicting interests of the patients, the insurer, and the hospital.

Despite these restraints on traditional decisionmaking, an increase in privatization presents opportunities for psychiatrists. Newer hospitals with substantial capital resources provide modern settings and technologies. Since most (though not all) hospital companies began as general hospital providers, they are well grounded in a "medical model" of organization that tends to preserve for physicians a major role in the provision of care and in clinical decisionmaking. Newly established hospitals, largely in the South and the West, where the population is growing, have increased their direct and indirect advertising to recruit psychiatrists; a survey by the APA showed that the majority of psychiatrists who relocated to another state are in the under-40 age group, apparently following financial incentives associated with increasing demand for psychiatrists in areas experiencing industrial growth. The number of psychiatrists citing a private psychiatric specialty hospital as their primary work site roughly tripled during the decade 1980 to 1990.

CHAPTER 5 _____

A Study of Psychiatric Services: An Overview

In the 1980s, the significant increase in the amount of both general medical and psychiatric health care provided by proprietary institutions has sparked debate between those who believe for-profit management results in care that is given more efficiently and is equal in quality to that given by nonprofit or public facilities and those who believe that the profit motive interferes with socially desirable concerns (Dorwart and Schlesinger, 1988). What has been lacking in the debate, thus far, is a database of sufficient breadth and detail documenting clinical and administrative practices, as well as economic and demographic features affecting those practices. In conducting a national study of psychiatric inpatient facilities, we attempted to fill this gap in 1988 (Dorwart, et al. 1991). Three primary research questions were addressed. First, does the ownership form of a hospital (for-profit, private nonprofit or public) influence the diagnostic mix, financial mix, referral sources, staffing practices, or services provided? Second, is type of hospital (specialty versus psychiatric unit within a general hospital) related to services provided, patient mix, or staffing practices? Third, how does competition within a service area affect variables such as services provided, diagnostic mix, financial mix, staffing practices, and marketing practices? We considered, as well, the possible effects of privatization on innovation in the delivery of mental health services. The following section is a brief summary of the methods and procedures used in the conduct of our study, the National Mental Health Facilities study.

OVERVIEW OF STUDY

In September 1988, a 200-item survey was distributed to administrators of all nonfederal psychiatric hospitals in the United States, including community mental health centers with inpatient units of more than forty beds, and to a 75 percent random sample of psychiatric units in nonfederal general hospitals. The sample was cross-checked with listings from the NIMH Master Facility File, the American Hospital Association (AHA), and the National Association of Private Psychiatric Hospitals (NAPPH). The resulting 1,604 facilities were sent questionnaires by New England Research Institute, Inc. and the Center for Health Policy (now Center for Social Policy) at the John F. Kennedy School of Government, Harvard University. Topic areas addressed in the questionnaire were: access to care; quality of care; economic performance; continuity of care; systems relationships and institutional linkages; organizational control; and values and perceptions of hospital administrators. Of the initial 1,604 questionnaires sent out, 1,551 were potentially available for participation. Of these 1,551 facilities, 915 (57 percent) returned questionnaires eligible for analysis. These facilities were divided into six categories: public psychiatric hospitals, public general hospital psychiatric units, nonprofit psychiatric hospitals, nonprofit general hospital psychiatric units, for-profit psychiatric hospitals, and for-profit general hospital psychiatric units. The response rates among the six facility categories ranged from 78 percent for public specialty hospitals to 38 percent for for-profit specialty hospitals.

The comparatively low response rate for for-profit psychiatric hospitals prompted a comparison of selected responses received from these participants with data from the NIMH (1986) and the NAPPH (1988). Comparison on several indices, including diagnostic mix of patients, source of revenue, staffing ratios, size of facility, and occupancy rate, indicated that the sample of private psychiatric hospitals in the current study was representative of the broader population of hospitals in this category.

It became apparent that the study could benefit from incorporation of additional data about mental health providers outside of institutions, such as community mental health centers and individual office-based practitioners. We therefore undertook two special studies. First, collection of data from CMHCs was undertaken by Robin Clark, Ph.D., who chose to work with us on the CMHC special study. The National Council of Community Mental Health Centers agreed to collaborate with us and Clark by incorporating our data collection needs into their annual survey of centers.

Second, in 1988, the same year the hospital survey questionnaires were distributed, the APA sponsored a national survey of psychiatrists' professional activities. We obtained permission to use these data in our service area analysis. This required completing data coding of the APA data and an additional special step to create geographic markers for the APA data so that they could, eventually, be matched to ours by state, county, and metropolitan area. The CMHC and APA studies are described in Chapter 6 of this book.

MAJOR FINDINGS

Behavior, by Ownership Form and Hospital Type

Ownership form and hospital type of the facilities responding to our survey of psychiatric hospitals were examined independently and interactively and were found to be significantly related to a number of clinical and administrative policies and practices. The following summarizes some of these findings.

Diagnostic mix. Previous studies of psychiatric hospitals have found that patients were selected for admission to private hospitals partly on the basis of ability to pay, but it was unclear whether, within ownership categories, specialty and general hospitals treated a different mix of patients based on diagnosis. Nor was it clear whether psychiatric units of general hospitals would follow the same ownership-related patterns in admitting patients as did psychiatric specialty hospitals.

The current study found that public hospitals, particularly specialty hospitals, are more likely to treat patients with schizophrenia than are private hospitals (see Table 5.1). Schizophrenia is usually a disorder with early onset, one that is commonly chronic and recurrent, and is often associated with marked disability in psychosocial functioning. These patients are costlier if for no other reason than their considerable length of stay, which is two to three times that of patients with affective disorders or chemical dependencies. These case-mix differences suggest that private facilities are specializing in disorders that usually respond to short-term treatment. Among specialty hospitals, those privately owned treat twice the proportion of patients with a diagnosis of depression as do publics. For schizophrenia and depression, the mix of patients in inpatient psychiatric units of general hospitals, regardless of ownership, looks more like that of private than public psychiatric hospitals.

Specialty hospitals serve a greater proportion of patients with disorders of childhood and adolescence than do general hospitals, and among

Table 5.1
Diagnoses of Patients Admitted to Nonfederal U.S. Psychiatric Hospitals and Units in 1988[a]

	Percent of Patients[b]												
	Specialty Hospital						General Hospital Unit						ANOVA	
	Public (N=172)[c]		Nonprofit (N=63)		For-Profit (N=106)[c]		Public (N=115)[c]		Nonprofit (N=411)[c]		For-Profit (N=36)			
Diagnosis	Mean	SD	Mean	SD	Mean	SD	Mean	SD	Mean	SD	Mean	SD	F	df
Schizophrenia	44.2$_a$	16.7	21.5$_{b,c}$	16.0	18.1$_c$	20.3	29.4$_d$	17.9	23.5$_b$	15.6	21.7$_{b,c,d}$	14.7	48.37^d	5, 896
Depression	18.2$_a$	10.0	34.0$_{b,d}$	18.5	34.7$_d$	21.0	27.2$_b$	14.7	35.2$_d$	18.9	26.7$_{a,b,d}$	20.0	26.20^d	5, 898
Substance abuse	13.1$_{a,d}$	15.0	13.1$_{a,d}$	13.4	16.8$_a$	19.5	13.8$_{a,d}$	14.6	10.5$_d$	13.5	15.9$_{a,d}$	14.7	3.96^e	5, 898
Disorders of childhood and adolescence	4.4$_a$	6.3	10.0$_d$	13.5	15.6$_b$	17.6	5.1$_a$	6.4	5.1$_a$	9.4	8.0$_{a,d}$	10.1	21.76^d	5, 897
Other[f]	20.2$_a$	12.7	21.6$_{a,d}$	13.5	14.6$_c$	11.4	24.3$_{a,d}$	12.8	25.9$_d$	14.9	28.0$_d$	22.0	20.67^d	5, 891

[a]Data are unweighted with respect to number of patients represented by each reporting institution.
[b]Matching subscripts indicate nonsignificant differences. Means in same row that do not share a subscript differ at $p \leq 0.05$ (Tukey's Studentized range test).
[c]Numbers vary slightly for each analysis.
[d]$p \leq 0.0001$.
[e]$p \leq 0.002$.
[f]For example, personality disorders, anxiety disorders, and organic brain syndrome.

specialty hospitals, proprietary hospitals treat the largest proportion, followed by nonprofit and public hospitals respectively. These types of disorders have long been characterized by unmet need for inpatient care, suggesting that an influx of private capital may be filling the gap.

Financial mix. What is most notable about the data on source of revenue is that both public and private hospitals receive substantial proportions of total revenues from a mix of sources (see Table 5.2). This suggests that government-owned hospitals may operate under some of the same conditions of reimbursement as private hospitals. Public specialty hospitals, often perceived by policymakers as financed by the states, actually received over half their payments from third-party payers such as Medicaid, Medicare, and commercial insurers. Psychiatric units within public general hospitals receive over three-quarters of their revenues from third-party sources. Conversely, private hospitals receive a significant proportion of their funding from public sources despite restrictions on Medicaid payments for adult patients aged 21–24 in specialty hospitals. Among private nonprofit specialty hospitals and units of general hospitals, over one-third of all revenues come from public auspices under either state grants, or Medicaid and Medicare. For-profit hospitals receive one-quarter of their revenues from these sources.

Staffing patterns and ratios. Using data collected in earlier NIMH surveys for comparison, the current data show a substantial reduction in the ratio of patients to staff over the past ten years in both public and private facilities. The changes have been greatest in state and county hospitals where, historically, staffing was the least adequate. Nonprofit psychiatric hospitals still have a lower patient-psychiatrist ratio (12.8 including staff and attending psychiatrists) than do public (31.7) or for-profit (18.5) psychiatric hospitals. Patient-psychiatrist ratios are lower, overall, in psychiatric units of general hospitals than in specialty hospitals, regardless of ownership. Among general hospitals, nonprofit facilities have the lowest ratio (9.3) as compared to public (11.1) or for-profit (13.1) units. Patient-staff ratios for all clinical staff are presented in Table 5.3.

Monitoring treatment. Regulators and payers increasingly examine patterns of practice in psychiatry and other areas of medicine to determine behaviors that improve both quality of care and cost effectiveness. Aftercare is an especially important dimension of treatment. Appropriate mental health care requires a successful transition from care as an inpatient to living in the community, typically with the support of some aftercare services. In practice, patients at a vulnerable time are often "lost" from any supportive services. The hospitals surveyed for this study differed significantly both in the extent to which they viewed aftercare as their respon-

Table 5.2
Source of Revenues for Nonfederal U.S. Psychiatric Hospitals and Units in 1988

	Percent of Revenue[a]												ANOVA	
Source of Revenue	Specialty Hospital						General Hospital Unit							
	Public (N=159)[b]		Nonprofit (N=64)		For-Profit (N=109)[b]		Public (N=113)[b]		Nonprofit (N=406)[b]		For-Profit (N=35)[b]			
	Mean	SD	Mean	SD	Mean	SD	Mean	SD	Mean	SD	Mean	SD	F	df
Insurance[c]	13.3_a	15.8	53.8_b	27.4	68.3_c	26.7	32.4_d	22.8	43.1_e	18.1	$48.7_{b,c}$	15.4	108.30^d	5, 875
Medicare	17.9_a	18.8	$13.5_{a,b}$	10.9	11.1_b	12.3	$19.8_{a,c}$	12.0	25.7_d	12.9	$27.2_{c,d}$	13.4	27.44^d	5, 882
Medicaid	22.7_a	23.3	10.0_b	16.8	9.6_b	21.9	24.6_a	19.9	20.0_a	14.5	$16.2_{a,b}$	16.9	12.72^d	5, 882
State government and contracts	35.1_a	40.6	13.0_b	24.5	$3.6_{c,d}$	9.9	$11.2_{b,c}$	21.5	2.8_d	6.9	$2.0_{b,c,d}$	4.7	59.42^d	5, 880
Patient and other	$9.6_{a,c}$	14.0	$7.0_{a,b}$	8.0	5.5_b	6.7	11.5_c	12.6	$8.0_{a,b}$	7.7	$6.6_{a,b,c}$	7.3	5.22^d	5, 879

[a] Matching subscripts indicate nonsignificant differences. Means in same row that do not share a subscript differ at $p \leq 0.05$ (Tukey's Studentized range test).
[b] Numbers vary slightly for each analysis.
[c] Blue Cross/Blue Shield, commercial insurance, and health maintenance organizations.
[d] $p \leq 0.0001$.

Table 5.3
Ratio of Patients to Full-Time Staff in Nonfederal U.S. Psychiatric Hospitals and Units in 1988

	Specialty Hospital									General Hospital Unit									ANOVA	
	Public			Nonprofit			For-Profit			Public			Nonprofit			For-Profit				
		Ratio[a,b]			Ratio[a,b]			Ratio[a,b]			Ratio[a,b]			Ratio[a,b]			Ratio[a,b]				
Staff	N^a	Mean	SD	N^a	Mean	SD	N^a	Mean	SD	N^a	Mean	SD	N^a	Mean	SD	N^a	Mean	SD	F	df
All psychiatrists	167	31.7_a	32.6	64	12.8_b	17.2	111	18.5_b	29.2	113	11.1_c	11.2	405	9.3_c	8.0	35	$13.1_{b,c}$	16.7	33.29^c	5, 889
Staff psychiatrists	165	32.0_a	32.6	52	21.6_c	26.7	77	31.6_c	29.0	71	10.1_b	11.0	235	15.5_b	14.1	13	16.0_c	14.2	16.07^c	5, 607
Private attending psychiatrists	—			43	$29.3_{a,b}$	32.7	93	33.1_a	48.4	62	$17.8_{b,c}$	15.7	360	15.9_c	19.6	32	$14.8_{b,c}$	17.2	9.31^c	5, 585
Psychologists	160	68.5_a	75.6	53	26.2_c	35.7	70	43.3_b	37.7	63	15.6_c	13.6	203	19.3_c	16.2	14	17.3_c	8.5	25.99^c	5, 557
Social workers	170	29.6_a	30.1	60	10.8_b	11.4	105	16.7_b	17.6	107	12.1_b	20.6	383	12.7_b	9.6	34	17.1_b	12.6	23.67^c	5, 853
Registered nurses	170	5.8_a	6.0	63	3.0_d	4.9	109	3.8_b	4.8	111	1.8_c	1.6	404	1.7_c	1.7	35	2.3_d	3.3	34.47^c	5, 886
L.P.N., mental health worker, other direct care provider	155	1.5_a	1.5	45	$1.5_{a,b}$	1.5	91	1.5_b	0.8	77	$1.6_{a,b}$	1.1	246	2.1_b	1.8	29	$2.0_{a,b}$	1.0	4.44^d	5, 637

[a]Based on responses greater than zero.
[b]Matching subscripts indicate nonsignificant differences. Means in same row that do not share a subscript differ at $p \leq 0.05$ (Tukey's Studentized range test).
[c]$p \leq 0.0001$.
[d]$p \leq 0.0005$.

sibility and in the efforts they devoted to following patients after discharge from the hospital.

Private hospitals rely heavily on office-based practitioners to provide postdischarge care (about 50 percent of private facilities as compared to 5 percent of public ones). Despite this practice, 72 percent of private nonprofit facilities and 65 percent of for-profit ones said they have a particular staff member or department whose primary responsibility is aftercare. Overall, about half (46 percent) of the hospitals reported following patients for one week or less, although 15 percent said they monitored patients' status for up to one year. Specialty facilities typically monitored patients longer than did general hospital psychiatric units; nearly half (47 percent) of the nonprofit specialty hospitals monitored patient status for six to twelve months, compared with 14 percent of the nonprofit general hospitals.

Community services. With the increased privatization of care, some observers have predicted that private for-profit hospitals, particularly those owned by multihospital systems, would be less likely than nonprofits to respond to community needs. Presumably this lack of responsiveness would be due to a drive to maximize profits and because the controlling corporate body of the institution was located outside the community. Such hospitals might discontinue unprofitable services, avoid working with preexisting public providers, or fail to provide services of community-wide benefit, such as medical education or emergency services. Results of our study generally confirmed that for-profit hospitals show less involvement in potentially unprofitable services. For-profit hospitals are less likely to provide emergency services than are nonprofit or public hospitals. General hospitals, regardless of ownership, are more likely to provide this service than psychiatric hospitals. Case-management for chronically ill patients, a service that is unprofitable because it is often not covered by insurance, was offered by 50 percent of public specialty hospitals, 39 percent of nonprofit facilities, and 7 percent of for-profits surveyed.

Accepting Referrals. Another measure of community involvement and responsiveness is the extent to which privately controlled general hospitals and private psychiatric hospitals accommodate the public sector market by accepting referrals from traditional public sector sources such as social welfare agencies and the courts, and by entering into contractual arrangements with state and local governments. This issue of whether community needs will be met arises from concern about the effects of the profit motive on the quality and accessibility of mental health services. It also arises from the debate over whether general hospitals should take a larger role in serving the public sector. Those advocating that they do so argue that general hospitals are the logical "linchpin" in the psychiatric service system because of their geographic accessibility to patients and providers, and because less stigma is felt by patients and their families when admission is to a community hospital rather than to a state institution (Fisher, et al., 1992). Furthermore, general hospitals are seen as having the advantages of an established emergency capability.

The current data show contracting to provide services more common than acceptance of referrals as a mechanism to provide access to the public sector. Of the 622 private hospitals surveyed, 265 (42.5 percent) had contracted with government at some level in the previous year, while referrals from public agencies accounted for 20 percent or more of all admissions in only 154 hospitals (24.7 percent). The two practices appeared to be related; 86 hospitals (13.8 percent) both contracted and accepted large numbers of public referrals. Of those hospitals which had a high proportion of public sector referrals, 55 percent also contracted to provide services, while one-third of contracting hospitals also took high levels of referrals. Forty-six percent of all private hospitals surveyed, however, neither contracted nor accepted significant numbers of referrals.

Among privately-owned facilities, nonprofit psychiatric hospitals were more likely to engage in contractual relationships than were psychiatric units in nonprofit general hospitals, for-profit specialty hospitals, or psychiatric units of for-profit general hospitals. Ownership form and hospital type were not significant predictors of referral involvement. However, competition and percentage of unemployment in the state were both negative predictors of contracting. Hospital administrators' perceptions of competition were also negatively associated with involvement; the higher the level of perceived competition, the lower the rate of referrals accepted from public sector agencies.

Competition and Ownership Form

One of the primary features of the increasingly privatized mental health care system in the United States has been an increase in competition for patients. Proprietary institutions are, by their nature, thought to be focussed on "the bottom line" and, therefore, strive to maintain a high proportion of insured to underinsured and uninsured patients. If this is the case, it is likely that as the number of proprietaries increases, nonprofit and public institutions will be forced to treat a higher proportion of the underinsured and uninsured than they had previously, thus increasing the burden on the voluntary sector. At the same time, nonprofit institutions have traditionally relied on cross-subsidizing to fund treatment of less well-insured patients; if the insured are cared for by for-profit facilities, the nonprofits may be forced to treat fewer of the less fortunate and to compete more actively for insured patients whose fees allow them to fulfill their public mission. Public facilities are also potentially affected. While the impact of competition on public facilities may be less, or indirect, the political and economic climate created by privatization and deregulation in the last decade has introduced a public expectation that government-sponsored institutions should more closely pursue the fiscal restraints of the private sector.

The current study examined the impact of competition on the behavior of hospitals as a function of ownership form and hospital type. Two measurements of competition were used. One was a questionnaire item asking hospital administrators the extent to which they had to compete with other institutions in their service area for new patients in the previous year. The second measurement was a rating of market concentration assigned to each hospital based on the Herfindahl index, which measures the number of similar institutions in a given area (White and Chirikos, 1988). The current study examined patients' access to services, and the delivery of care as a function of ownership form and type of hospital (general versus specialty) under varying degrees of competition (low to high).

The Herfindahl Index. The extent of competition faced by each facility was measured using the Herfindahl index (HI) of market concentration, a measure of competition used frequently by economists. In our study, it provided an objective economic index of competition as a framework within which to view administrators' own ratings of perceived competition and their related decisions within the last year. As compared to several other indices of market concentration, the HI takes into account both size and number of facilities in a given market area. Using the Herfindahl index, scores ranging between 0 and 1 were assigned to each facility. A score of 1 indicates a highly concentrated market in which a single facility serves the entire service area. This monopoly, obviously, represents low competition. A score of 0 indicates low concentration; in other words, a highly saturated market where each facility is in heavy competition for its relatively small portion of the total market.

Interestingly, administrators' ratings of competition matched Herfindahl index ratings for their area in a surprisingly large number of cases. Administrators' judgments in for-profit general hospitals matched Herfindahl ratings 60 percent of the time. Public general hospital administrators' judgments corresponded to Herfindahl ratings 33 percent of the time. For-profit and nonprofit specialty hospitals were most likely to overestimate competition, while public psychiatric units of general hospitals underestimated competition most often.

Access. Access to care was measured by us in several ways: the limitation of access was indicated if patients were being screened for insurance coverage, or if marginally profitable services were being eliminated; the promotion of access was measured by the use of direct marketing, the addition of new services, and the provision of specialized services (e.g., geriatric, eating disorders, alcohol and substance abuse). The degree to which hospitals promoted access was shown as well by the amount of uncompensated care and care at reduced charges offered.

The limitation of access through eliminating marginally profitable services was found to be a response by all institutions under high versus low competition. However, as might be expected, the most marked response was by for-profit facilities.

All facilities reported a lower proportion of revenues from Medicaid-funded patients as competition increased, a measure of screening practice. However, for-profit specialty hospitals exhibited a higher gradient in this effect; that is, they appear to be more sensitive than other institutions to this variable under conditions of greater competition. Overall, public general hospitals' psychiatric units had the largest percent of uncollected fees at all three levels of competition (31 percent at low, 22 percent at high). However, nonprofit specialty facilities showed the sharpest decline from low to high competition (23 percent to 6 percent). These figures suggest that the mission and capabilities of nonprofit providers may be changing dramatically as a function of increased privatization and competition. These findings seem to confirm the theory that where there are few hospitals in a community, those that exist feel an obligation to serve the needy. With increased competition they may not only be unable to subsidize the poor, but may expect the obligation to be shared.

Promotion of access through direct marketing and the addition of services to attract new patients was reported by all facilities (including those owned by government) when competition was high. For-profit facilities pursue these activities more adamantly than others.

We found wide variation in our national study in the percentage of patients' charges uncollected. Mean proportions of uncompensated inpatient care (for specialty and general hospitals combined) ranged from 9 percent in proprietary hospitals to 35 percent in public hospitals. This ownership-related pattern is consistent with the findings of previous studies, although it is notable that differences between for-profit and private nonprofit hospitals are more pronounced for specialty than general hospitals and for outpatient than inpatient services. It is also striking that public psychiatric hospitals offer a relatively small amount of uncompensated outpatient care, suggesting that there is a fairly sharp split in administrators' sense of mission as provider of last resort between outpatient and inpatient care.

We also asked administrators to report the proportion of patients who received care at reduced charges (excluding discounts negotiated with insurers or other contractual allowances). We did this because we wanted to capture the hospitals' total response to care of the poor. Hospitals that offer care at reduced charge to low income patients (who are less likely than others to pay) will thus report a lower cost for uncompensated care than will those who do not reduce charges, even if they are treating the same number of nonpaying patients. Despite these apparent similarities, it is important to recognize that reduced charges capture a rather different aspect of access than does aggregate uncompensated care. As noted earlier, the latter may primarily reflect inability to discharge patients who outstay their insurance coverage. Reduced charges, on the other hand, tend to increase access for patients without insurance or for those whose insurance requires substantial copayments for mental health care and who might therefore be unable to seek care at full charge.

It is clear that the trends associated with privatization combine to reduce (1) the total volume of uncompensated care, (2) admissions for the uninsured, and (3) the capacity to meet unexpected increases in demand for uncompensated care. Privatization also increases the propensity of hospitals to transfer patients for financial reasons. But some of these reductions in access may be offset by the growing number of mental health providers and the shift of care to general hospitals, both of which should increase the geographic accessibility of mental health care, especially for patients who do have some insurance.

Delivery of care. The delivery of care was measured with three questions related to staffing practices: the ratio of patients to psychiatrists, the reduction of non-physician clinical staff in the previous year, and the reduction of administrative staff in the previous year. Again, for-profit institutions showed the most dramatic response to competitive environments. They are the most likely to reduce nonphysician clinical and administrative staff. They are also most likely to reduce the patient-physician ratio. This shift appears, however, to be "corrective," making the staffing in for-profits more comparable to nonprofit and public institutions when they face high competition conditions. Nonprofits maintain a relatively stable patient-physician ratio across levels of competition, but they also report a reduction in administrative staff and nonphysician clinicians under high competition.

Ownership and Innovation

One of the arguments for privatization is that the private sector fosters greater responsibility to consumer demand and therefore more innovation. In contrast, the public sector is often said by its critics to operate in an inflexible and bureaucratic mode. We examine briefly here our observations of the relationship between ownership form and innovation in the services provided based on our study of psychiatric facilities.

There is a broad presumption in American policymaking that, all else equal, it is desirable to foster social institutions that are adaptive, flexible, and innovative. Indeed, some observers attribute much of the prevailing crisis of legitimacy in government to the perception that public institutions have become too inflexible. "The ability of Western governments to surmount the current crisis depends on what might be called their 'learning capacity.' A government must be able to recognize the existence of a new problem for which past solutions or incremental adjustments are inadequate . . . " (Merritt and Merritt, 1985, p. 10).

The goal of establishing a more flexible and responsive delivery system than that provided in the past by government is behind efforts to further privatize health and social services. Although it is sometimes acknowledged that organizations providing these services could in principle become too sensitive to change, resulting in interruptions in the continuity of care, there is a broad presumption that these service delivery systems are more often inadequately responsive to changing external conditions and needs. Claims that contracting with private nonprofit or for-profit agencies would increase innovation and responsiveness are based on only a vague sense of how exactly organizational structure shapes behavior.

The case for privatization remains ill-defined in part because the dynamic of organizational behavior can be quite complicated. Concepts of "innovation," "responsiveness," and "flexibility" are themselves inexact and difficult to define. This makes them easy to endorse as a goal, but the attainment of the goal is difficult to evaluate. This complexity is conveyed by the number of distinctions that are typically drawn in the literature between types of innovation. One distinction involves passive versus active—the difference between responding to external changes and generating new changes, sometimes referred to as the differences between innovation and invention. A second distinction is one between magnitude and timing. An organization may be viewed as more responsive than another if it reacts to problems to either a greater extent or with greater alacrity.

The same factors that encourage invention also encourage innovation, since as an organization implements any new service or technique of service delivery it in some sense "reinvents" the innovation. This is particularly true for health and human services, where the nature of service delivery depends greatly on idiosyncratic characteristics of the particular clients receiving the services. The distinction between speed and magnitude of response is more salient in principle. There is a public interest in ensuring more rapid adjustment to changing conditions (whatever the eventual new equilibrium) but not for preferring a larger reaction to change. Here too, however, there is likely to be a positive correlation between the two aspects of responsiveness, since the larger the desired long-term response by the organizations, the larger will be its short-term response to any changes. For purposes of our conceptual discussion, we will focus on speed of response (Golden, 1991).

We assume that many of the key observations and resource allocation decisions are made by employees in a decentralized manner. Central authorities shape the overall policies of the organization, but have only limited control over implementation of these policies. This pattern of organization is common to many health and human service agencies, particularly those in which there is substantial government payment for services to clients. Because service allocations depend on the varied needs of individual clients, and it is costly for the central authorities to closely monitor service delivery, providers are often trained and disposed to act under professional norms that guide their actions in these unsupervised settings.

During the past decade, the types of inpatient mental health care being delivered changed considerably. In part this reflected increased attention to particular disorders or groups of mentally ill, including the elderly, children and adolescents, those with eating disorders, and with problems of substance abuse. This led to the development of new services targeted to these groups. It also encouraged the creation of contracts and referral agreements with other service providers who specialized in these populations.

A second major source of innovation came from changes in the ways that mental health services were purchased. Historically, hospitals had attracted patients by competing for the physicians who treated them, assuming patients would go where their doctors led. But increasingly over the past decade, hospitals have directly marketed themselves to potential individual clients, to employers who operate work site-based mental health care programs (typically referred to as employee assistance plans, or EAPs) and to insurance plans that have pre-enrolled populations (Dorwart and Epstein, 1992). At the same time, purchasers of services have grown more cost conscious, adopting payment systems that encouraged treatment of shorter duration and the creation of case management programs to limit unnecessary care (Schlesinger, 1989).

Data on Hospital Innovativeness

Our national survey of psychiatric hospitals explored some of the relationships between ownership and organizational responsiveness, often referred to simply as "innovativeness." In particular, we examined the influence of ownership—a key proxy in the analysis of privatization—on taking initiatives to make services more flexible and responsive to the needs of a diverse population.

For purposes of this analysis, we assessed the amount of innovation/ responsiveness at a facility by its adoption of a set of services and management techniques that were in the process of being implemented at the time the hospital was surveyed. These innovations were aggregated into a set of indices and used as dependent variables in a regression model. Facility ownership and the extent of competition that it faced were included as independent variables in these regressions, with the coefficients on these variables measuring the relative rate of adoption of these innovations.

Three separate indices were calculated. (Separate analyses were also conducted on each component. The results were roughly comparable to those discussed for the aggregate indices.) The first index measured the addition of any of four innovative services—treatment units for children/adolescents, geriatric psychiatry, eating disorders, and substance abuse. The second index combined four emerging management practices oriented primarily to privately insured clients: direct marketing to patients, encouraging short-term treatment, entering into contracts with insurance plans, and forming contracts with EAPs. The third index combined innovative management practices oriented primarily to publicly financed patients. These were case management for the chronically mentally ill, contracts with nursing homes, and contracts with home health agencies. We report the general results below.

Several of our findings were striking. It appears that ownership does affect response to changing conditions, but in ways that are different from and more complex than suggested by the standard case for privatization.

There is no evidence that private facilities are inherently more innovative than are government agencies, when both types of facilities operate as monopolies. But for at least some innovations, the relative responsiveness of private agencies is quite sensitive to the amount of competition that they face. As competition intensifies, both private nonprofit and for-profit agencies become significantly more likely to adopt new services as well as management techniques oriented to privately-financed clients. (The effect of competition on innovations oriented to public financed clients is much weaker.) In extremely competitive settings, both types of private facilities appear more innovative than government agencies facing comparable levels of competition.

For-profit agencies do appear to be more responsive to competitive pressures than do their private nonprofit counterparts. For the diffusion of services and management techniques targeted to privately-financed clients, these differences were statistically significant. However, the case that for-profit agencies are inherently more innovative than their private nonprofit counterparts receives little support. In noncompetitive environments, private nonprofit firms appear significantly more responsive to change than are for-profits. Only in the most competitive settings do for-profit agencies ever appear more innovative, and then only for the adoption of new services, not for adopting new management techniques.

Implications for Understanding Privatization

These findings, taken together with other aspects of our research, are suggestive of some effects of privatization that appear to have policy implications. As noted earlier, the prevailing view of nonprofit ownership is that it encourages organizations to behave in a manner that is in some sense intermediate between private for-profit and government agencies. This view received some support from our studies on innovation. The extent of response of private nonprofit firms to competitive pressures was larger than that of their government counterparts, while smaller than that of comparable for-profit service providers. The use of patient satisfaction instruments and formalized referral arrangements was less frequent in nonprofit agencies than in for-profit, but more common than in government facilities.

We find that ties to the community play a critical role in influencing when nonproprietary organizations respond more quickly than do proprietary firms to changing conditions. The market is in some cases an inefficient and incomplete channel for conveying preferences. To the extent that firms directly internalize these in their agency mission, or are tied to alternative sources of information from the community, they may prove more responsive to changing external conditions.

Our results also raise some serious questions about the fundamental assumption underlying privatization—that private agencies are inherently more adaptable than are government agencies. They suggest that in noncompetitive circumstances, government agencies will in fact be more innovative. Some aspects of bureaucratization are apparently positively associated with innovation. The spread of some innovations is encouraged by oversight from state officials, which may also serve to convey information about new practices that are not readily communicated in noncompetitive circumstances.

If contracting with private (particularly for-profit) monopolists almost certainly impedes rather than enhances innovation, the question remains of whether *on average* privatization increases responsiveness. In our study, private firms have higher rates of use of management innovations than do government agencies, but the reverse is true for instituting new services. In practice, deciding whether (and with whom) to privatize services is a complicated question. Private providers behave differently under different levels of competition. They may, moreover, decide to locate in dissimilar markets, so that they necessarily face different levels of competition. In this survey, administrators in for-profit agencies reported a perceived level of competition that was almost 20 percent higher than that reported by their counterparts in nonprofit settings. They may in fact be operating in more competitive markets, but they may simply perceive higher levels of competition. At the reported levels of competition perceived by the average for-profit provider, they tend to adopt innovative services more rapidly than do nonprofit agencies, although they still lag behind on the diffusion of management innovations.

The Influence of Competition and Ownership on Access to Care

The major concern about the effects of privatization in mental health services, which we have described and analyzed in this and earlier chapters, is maintaining access to care, especially for poor patients. Privatization has affected the traditional role played by private hospitals, which have long provided the bulk of the care needed by those without private insurance. Many private hospitals continue to provide this care, sometimes at substantial cost to the facility. This legacy of community service appears strongest, for a variety of reasons, among general hospitals (Stevens, 1989). First, these hospitals often were established at a time when philanthropy paid for a good deal of their capital needs (Marmor, et al., 1987). This created in both legal and social terms a "fiduciary relationship" between the hospital and the community in which it operated. Second, most of these hospitals received government funding under the 1946 Hill-Burton program. This carried with it an explicit requirement to care for indigent patients, a requirement that has been interpreted with greater breadth and enforced with greater vigor in recent years. Finally, many of these hospitals have important links to the community through their boards of directors. This may allow the community a certain amount of control, or at least some influence, over the facility's operation and policies. In contrast, the smaller number of private psychiatric hospitals are often located outside local neighborhoods and are less likely to have strong ties to the community. They also have no obligation to community service based on public or philanthropic donations.

How willing private facilities are to treat unprofitable patients may affect access for the mentally ill who are inadequately insured and for those who must rely on government insurance. A larger number of the mentally ill than of those who have a physical illness are without private insurance. Not all private health insurance policies cover mental illness and when they do, they may have restrictive ceilings on psychiatric hospitalization. Even those who are employed and insured may have inadequate coverage for psychiatric treatment. The more severely and chronically mentally ill are likely to lose their jobs, and with them, their employment-based insurance. Although state-owned hospitals have historically treated much of this latter population, the number of beds in these facilities has fallen by more than half since 1970, leaving private facilities often as the only source of care.

There are thus two distinct populations of the mentally ill whose access to care may be limited. The first are those without any third-party coverage. According to our national survey of psychiatric inpatient facilities, in 1988 roughly 8 percent of all patients were without any third-party coverage. In addition, a significant number of the patients covered by private insurance will exhaust their coverage for psychiatric hospital care each year and become uninsured. Hospitals will often try to discourage admissions of those without any insurance, and will discharge patients whose insurance has been exhausted. The first type of practice has been referred to as "creaming," the second as "dumping."

The second group are patients covered by government programs. As in the rest of the health care system, the Medicare and Medicaid programs are the primary sources of publicly financed care for the mentally ill, each paying for about 20 percent of all inpatient services, according to our survey. In addition, states also directly contract for mental health services from private hospitals. These contracts pay for just over 10 percent of all inpatient care, with somewhat more paid to specialty hospitals than to the psychiatric units of general hospitals. The willingness of hospitals to admit these patients will clearly depend in part on the generosity of the government program in paying for treatment, and these programs are typically not generous payers. But even if government programs paid rates comparable to those of private insurance, providers might avoid these patients because many are seriously ill and are more difficult to treat than the typical patient covered by employer-based insurance.

Accompanying, and to some extent creating, the growth of for-profit ownership of mental health care facilities has been an expansion of affiliations with multifacility systems (Schlesinger and Dorwart, 1984). These systems own or manage approximately 60 percent of the psychiatric specialty hospitals and 10 percent of the units in general hospitals (Redick, et al., 1989).

System affiliation may affect access for patients without private insurance in three ways (Schlesinger, et al., 1987). System affiliation transfers some of the control over the facility away from the local community to the system's central office (Ermann and Gabel, 1984). The extent to which this occurs appears to vary greatly from one system to the next—some are highly centralized, others relatively decentralized (Lindorff, 1992). Assuming that social constraints from the local community create pressure for care of unprofitable patients, any centralization of authority will reduce to some extent the willingness of the hospital to provide care to these patients.

A second and more favorable link between system affiliation and access involves the costs of care. Although there is little evidence that system-affiliated community hospitals are less expensive to operate than independent hospitals, there are certainly some economies of scale to be captured through group purchasing, use of management information systems, and the like (Renn, et al., 1985). To the extent that these economies operate effectively in providing psychiatric care at lower cost than in other hospitals, they might make system-affiliated hospitals significantly less expensive, allowing them to serve profitably at least some publicly-financed patients.

Finally, system affiliation gives the hospital access to resources and financial reserves that would otherwise be unavailable (Ermann and Gabel, 1984). Although no system is likely to subsidize large numbers of hospitals for any length of time, these fiscal advantages can certainly cover short-term shortfalls in revenues. This may allow individual hospitals to respond to temporary increases in the number of uninsured patients. Over the longer term, systems may be willing to support some institutions as "loss leaders," particularly if those facilities were engaged in teaching, research, or other activities that brought professional prestige to the other members of the system.

Gains in access were also reflected in some questions asked of administrators in the CMHC survey. Respondents were asked, "How difficult is it for the following types of mental health clients to gain admission to hospitals in your area?"—ranking that difficulty on a three-point scale. The question was asked for seriously mentally ill adults (separately for insured and uninsured) as well as for adolescents (insured and uninsured). As one moves from areas of low to high competition, access becomes easier for those with insurance, although access for uninsured patients becomes more difficult.

In sum, we have used the example of psychiatric hospitals to examine the influence of ownership and perceived competition on financial access to care. We found that ownership matters, but so does competition. Demand for psychiatric services (at least ambulatory care) is generally more sensitive to private insurance incentives and, as we demonstrate, also sensitive to the effects of competition. Despite the existence of a large public sector capacity for psychiatric hospital care, private hospitals offer significant amounts of uncompensated care and care at reduced charges; here, too, there are some ownership-related differences, with public general hospitals reporting the highest proportion of uncompensated care (24 percent of revenues). We also suggest that a growing private sector may place a greater burden on the public sector. Public sector facilities increasingly must treat a rising proportion of patients with severe, long-term mental illnesses (e.g., schizophrenia), but they also must rely on public funding that responds to the economic climate rather than the needs of their clientele.

CHAPTER 6_____

Privatization and Its Effects on CMHCs and Psychiatrists

In preceding chapters, we have described the development of the public and private mental health care systems with special emphasis on psychiatric hospitals and the financing of services. We have seen how there has been a dramatic shift in recent years from reliance on public funds and facilities to the use of third party insurance and private hospitals for providing inpatient psychiatric care. We have also noted how the philosophy of deinstitutionalization and the federal mandate for community mental health centers led to diversification of the locations of care, an increasing mix of organizations providing services, and changes in the patterns of practice. These trends have had mixed results in improving access to care for those in need of treatment, bringing increased access for those with insurance and decreased access for those without it. In Chapter 7, we will illustrate these changes with specific examples of how one community mental health care system developed and changed under the influence of privatization. In Chapter 8, we will discuss how in our view the mental health care system in the future must become more highly integrated with other health and social systems than it is at present.

In this chapter, we examine some of the effects of privatization on the delivery of community-based mental health services. In addition to elaborating on earlier discussions of the effects of privatization and competition on access to care and on institutional behavior, we also examine their effects on community mental health agencies (known at their inception as community mental health centers) and on psychiatrists' private practice patterns. We then discuss how privatization affects the relationship of state mental health authorities to community mental health agencies (CMHAs) as they rely increasingly on contracts to purchase services from private mental health providers rather than providing those services under state auspices. We conclude by outlining the major responses to competition adopted by providers of mental health care.

CMHCs and Privatization

The Federal Community Mental Health Center program, launched in the early 1960s during the Kennedy administration, represented the elevation of mental health policy to what Lynn (1982) has called the "high game" of public policy management: i.e., a concern of presidents, cabinet officials, high courts, and prominent public figures. In an expansive period for health and welfare programs nationally, a categorical approach supported by single-issue advocacy groups succeeded in establishing a federal role, albeit a relatively small one, in the direct provision of mental health services.

According to Lynn, the "high game" involves major policy decisions and establishes overall missions and mandates in a substantive policy area. The reform movement aspects of the legislation that introduced the concept of community mental health services resulted in part from the impact of high-level public policy decisions in Congress, at the NIMH, and in the courts. In Lynn's game metaphor for analyzing public policy management, the high-game action seeks to answer the question: "Is there a need for government action at all? If so, what is its purpose?" The "middle game" involves deciding what the role will be and the "low game" determines how programs will be organized and administered at the operational level.

But historically, mental health policy has been a middle game of state officials or a low game of state hospital superintendents, county and municipal officials, and mental health department administrators. Of the middle game, Lynn observes: "This is the predominant game for political executives, as well as the bread-and-butter game for legislators. . . . Debate is about results—that is, the effectiveness and efficiency of governmental actions—about the fairness, appropriateness and consequences of distributional effects, about administrative competence and about costs." This orientation toward more business-like operations can be seen in the evaluation of CMHCs.

A national survey of CMHCs by Woy, et al. (1981) of the NIMH found a continuation of trends detected earlier by Naierman, et al. (1978) in a study of a cohort of CMHCs ten years after initial funding, namely: (1) a changing mix of funding, once temporary federal support ended, toward increased state support and an increase in services reimbursed by third parties; and (2) a gradual shift in service mix and priorities away from providing services to all who needed them toward an increasing emphasis on services to those who could pay for them. Inpatient, outpatient, and emergency services were increased while partial hospitalization, home visits, and consultation and education—services not usually paid for by insurance—were cut back.

Woy, et al. found that the greatest growth was in emergency and outpatient services rather than inpatient services because only about 10 percent of CMHCs have inpatient facilities. They believe the changes toward insured services reflect a conservative approach to their funding dilemmas. These changes were more pronounced for older centers which had "graduated" from the eight-year federal funding period than for those still being funded.

An earlier study of this same cohort of CMHCs by Weiner, et al. (1979) suggested that the centers were dividing into two main groups, one publicly and the other privately funded. Woy, et al. agree that the crucial variable distinguishing the two groups was their degree of dependence on federal funding, but they see the differences between the publicly and privately oriented groups as sometimes indistinct: for example, some centers have a 50-50 public/private revenue base. They are not able to explain why some centers move away from the ideal CMHC model and others do not.

The *de facto* privatization of community mental health centers has evolved over more than twenty-five years since the inception of the federal program in 1963 that created a national network of local centers (see discussion in Chapter 2). The original goals of the community mental health center plan were to establish local centers serving defined geographic catchment areas and to provide a set of basic or core services for each community. The federal funding for the centers was seen as "seed money" that was to be phased out after a period of five to eight years (Foley and Sharfstein, 1983). Only about half as many centers (roughly 800) were created as were originally planned to provide services to communities most in need. Many different organizational models evolved and when the federal funding ended, centers employed different strategies to finance their work. Some centers diversified into primarily privately oriented agencies relying on third-party reimbursable services from a variety of funding streams. These centers often survived or even thrived at the expense of abandoning programs for the severely mentally ill or the poor. Other programs attempted to maintain their basic mission of serving the

entire community and providing services for patients regardless of their
ability to pay for treatment. Programs that provided non-reimbursable
services barely survived under poor financing or failed outright.

Today, the existing community mental health agencies provide most of
the institutional outpatient mental health treatment in the United States.
Much of the care is provided below cost and is uncompensated by
third-party payers. Such subsidized care is often supported under contracts
from the state mental health authorities and is stringently targeted to
priority client groups, such as the severely mentally ill. Although federal
start-up funds are no longer available for community mental health centers, their number has continued to increase to more than 2,200 today
(including private ones) largely because of the trend toward deinstitutionalization and the substituted reliance on outpatient treatment.

In order to understand better the role of CMHCs in the contemporary
mental health care system, including their responses to increasing competition, we carried out a national survey of centers in 1989, as indicated in
Chapter 5. The survey was conducted under the auspices of the Center for
Social Policy at the Kennedy School of Government at Harvard in collaboration with the National Council of Community Mental Health Centers.
The project director was Robin Clark, Ph.D. A total of 633 (59 percent)
out of 1,070 multiservice agencies and outpatient clinics returned questionnaires. Clark included federally sponsored centers in his study as well
as other community mental health clinics and used "agency" as a term for
all of them. Of agencies responding, 470 gave complete information for
our analysis. Nonprofit agencies comprised the majority (68 percent) of
respondents; 28 percent of respondents were publicly owned, and 4
percent were for-profit (Clark, and Dorwart, 1992).

We found that public and private community mental health agencies
were not significantly different in the total number of visits to their clinics
provided on average, although public agencies showed a tendency to
provide more below-cost (or subsidized) visits. This pattern of finding
similarities between private and public community mental health agencies
following a decade (the 1980s) of growing competition is similar to
another finding from our study of psychiatric hospitals, namely, that
proprietary and nonprofit hospitals tended to behave similarly in geographic areas where high competition existed. Not surprisingly, we found
that federally-initiated agencies provided more below-cost visits than
those started without federal sponsorship, even when we controlled the
size of the agency.

We discovered that community mental health agencies, in attempting
to cope with increasing competition and the pressures of privatization,

were adopting more stringent management practices. To increase efficiency, they contracted exclusively with one provider and improved their billing practices. They also sought ways to increase productivity, linking staff compensation to performance, encouraging the use of short-term therapies, and increasing their proportion of insured patients. Other common strategies were to diversify the services offered and to seek several sources of funding, including support from the community and from philanthropists. States often promoted privatization by contracting with private providers to purchase services. For example, in Massachusetts in 1991, the state transferred operational responsibility for its 110 mental-health clinics to private groups (Schroeder, 1992).

Although there were similarities, we also found numerous differences between public and private organizations. We surveyed 123 public and 335 private agencies. The public agencies were larger on average, reporting an average of thirty-seven as opposed to twenty-seven full-time equivalent staff and 20 percent more outpatient visits per year. However, outpatient revenue collected by the private agencies exceeded that of public ones, although both types reported providing the same number of below cost visits annually. As expected, private agencies reported receiving more of their revenues from client fees and from insurance revenues.

Public and private mental health agencies differed in the number of management strategies they employed aimed at reducing costs. Both public and private clinics felt pressure to adopt strategies to cope with competition, but the public agencies used somewhat different methods. Private agencies were significantly more likely than public ones to have used the following methods during the surveyed year: they increased their use of financial incentives to improve staff performance, increased the use of short-term therapy, increased emphasis on billable services, and increased efforts at verifying patients' finances and at collecting debts. Public agencies were more likely (or as likely) to do the following: divert insured patients to other providers, use group therapy, contract with outside agencies for billing or client tracking services, employ group purchasing of supplies or arrange for group health insurance, and participate in a local business/health coalition. Three-quarters of both public and private agencies reported working with other provider groups to attempt to influence government mental health policy (lobbying) and one-tenth of each category of agencies reported operating joint ventures with other provider agencies. Private agencies, on the other hand, were twice as likely as public agencies to seek funds from private charitable organizations or solicit the philanthropy of individual citizens.

Psychiatrists' Practices Respond to Change

In 1988–1989, in collaboration with the American Psychiatric Association's Committee on the Biographical Directory and Research on Professional Activities, we carried out a national survey of psychiatrists. When all responses were aggregated, we had roughly 19,500 subjects who responded to the questionnaire (for details of methods, see Dorwart, et al., 1992a). The median age of the respondents was 50 years and nearly 20 percent were women. The purpose of the survey was to learn more about psychiatrists and how aspects of practice, such as where they work, how they spend their time, and who they treat have changed from earlier periods. We were especially interested in how these practice trends relate to changes in mental health services delivery, brought about by privatization, medicalization, and specialization.

Although it is difficult to obtain an exact count of practicing psychiatrists in each state because states do not always record subspecialties, we have made an attempt to estimate these numbers here. Our data include psychiatrists in training, concentrated in medical schools and teaching hospitals. The estimates have a sizable margin of error, but are a rough guide to the distribution of practitioners.

Both the numbers of physicians and psychiatrists in the United States and the ratios of physicians and psychiatrists to overall population have steadily risen over the past forty years and, according to the American Medical Association, are expected to continue to increase. In 1970 the ratio of physicians per 100,000 population nationally was 148, and the ratio of psychiatrists was approximately 10. By 1988, the ratios had increased to 240/100,000 for all physicians and to 16.5/100,000 for psychiatrists, representing a roughly comparable two-thirds increase of psychiatrists and of physicians over this period. For psychiatrists, as for physicians generally, the distribution and rates of change in different regions, states, and metropolitan areas are uneven. For example, the ratios of active psychiatrists in our 1988 survey varied from 35 in the South Central region of the country, to 91 in the Pacific region, to 160 in the New England region. Our sample survey reveals that more than one-fourth of respondents practice in New York (15.7 percent) and California (13 percent). Six states together account for fewer than 1 percent of all psychiatrists in the study (Wyoming, North Dakota, South Dakota, Alaska, Idaho, and Montana). Since 1982, the number of psychiatrists per capita population increased in some states and declined in others, with growth following that of the population to western and southern regions of the country. Psychiatrists are disproportionately located in large urban areas.

One of the cardinal features of growth and change in psychiatry in the 1980s was a trend toward subspecialization. To measure this trend, we collected several kinds of information: data on training, certification, subspecialty interests of members, types of patients treated, and settings in which psychiatrists work.

Subspecialization has long been evident in the scientific and clinical pursuits of psychiatrists; however, recently there has been an accelerating trend toward formalization of subspecialties. The American Board of Psychiatry and Neurology (ABPN) was founded in 1934; the first subspecialty, child psychiatry, was approved by the ABPN in 1959. In April 1991, the ABPN gave its first examination to confer a certificate of added qualification in geropsychiatry, and several other subspecialties have requested similar status (e.g., addictionology, forensic psychiatry, administrative psychiatry, adolescent psychiatry, consultation/liaison psychiatry, and others).

Not surprisingly, we found that members often had organizational affiliations and clinical interests in subspecialties without having formal subspecialty fellowship training. An exception was child psychiatry where all those expressing interest (20 percent) had formal training and were members of the American Academy of Child and Adolescent Psychiatry. Among respondents who expressed interest in a subspecialty, some 30 percent treated adolescents, the elderly, alcohol abusers, or did consult-liaison for medical patients. Another 20 percent indicated administrative psychiatry and forensic psychiatry. Twelve percent expressed interest in research, and 3 percent of members had at least one year of formal research training. Many psychiatrists pursue their subspecialty interests through participation in specialty societies or organizations, as well as through training that is not necessarily full-time fellowship education.

We asked psychiatrists several questions about how they spend their time during a typical work week, including the type of settings in which they work, the functions they perform, the kinds of patients they see, and the modalities of treatment they commonly use. Psychiatrists work in a wide variety of settings and most work in more than one setting; the mean number of settings in 1988, as it was in 1982, was 2.3. For example, a psychiatrist might work half-time in a medical school, one-quarter time in a local community mental health center, maintain a part-time private office practice, and consult to a nursing home. In general, psychiatrists' practices have been characterized over the past twenty-five years by a predominance of private practice over other primary work settings and by a large and growing involvement in organization-based practice, such as hospitals and CMHAs.

In 1988, the proportion of psychiatrists reporting office-based private practice as their primary focus, i.e., the setting where they worked the greatest number of hours in a typical week, was 45 percent, compared to 58 percent in 1982. In addition, private practice remains the second most common secondary work setting, reported as such by 25 percent of respondents in 1988. The proportion of psychiatrists who work in private psychiatric hospitals showed the most significant change, rising from 3.7 percent in 1982 to 11 percent in 1988. The proportion working in free-standing clinics and HMOs rose only slightly, and the number working in medical schools or universities declined from 12.3 percent to 5.9 percent. The percent at work in HMOs was 1.4 percent—surprisingly few given the growth of HMOs during the 1980s. Just over 10 percent of all respondents indicated a state hospital as their primary work setting.

Another way of assessing the practice of psychiatrists is to look at the kinds of patients they treat. We asked respondents to describe by major diagnostic categories the patients they had seen in the preceding month. The largest category (25 percent) of patients seen had major affective disorders and 15 percent were classified as schizophrenic or had other psychotic disorders. Ten percent of all patients seen in a month sought treatment for substance abuse (drugs or alcohol), 10 percent had a personality disorder, and another 10 percent an anxiety disorder. Smaller numbers of patients sought help with childhood/developmental disorders (8 percent), adjustment problems (7 percent), or organic mental disorders (5 percent); the remainder had unclassified complaints. In general, psychiatrists' caseload is distributed across settings as follows: outpatient, 66 percent; inpatient, 30 percent; partial hospital, 4 percent. The average "caseload" for all psychiatrists in all settings is 62 patients.

In response to marked changes in the health-care system generally, as well as to evolving patterns of professional development, the practice of psychiatry is changing rapidly. One major change is the trend toward more services being provided in organized settings, including outpatient services of general hospitals. While the proportionate degree of involvement of psychiatrists in state hospitals and CMHCs remains roughly comparable to earlier periods, there has been an increase in work in general hospitals and in private psychiatric hospitals. This trend toward affiliations with hospitals is by no means new but the type of hospital has changed; according to Grob (1991), just after World War II two-thirds of psychiatrists were employed in state mental hospitals. Hospital affiliation reflects several underlying developments in mental health care. One reason for the trend toward hospital-based practice undoubtedly is the medicalization of psychiatry. We found that nearly 40 percent of respondents reported direct patient-care activities in inpatient settings, a majority commonly prescribed medications in treating their patients, and three-fourths reported some use of somatic therapies (or medical diagnostic assessments) in their practice. It is thus reasonable to say that the medical aspects of psychiatric practice are the *sine qua non* of psychiatrists' professional activities in the 1990s.

Another reason for the increase in hospital services by psychiatrists is the growth of private psychiatric hospitals during the 1980s, previously noted (Chapter 4), from fewer than 10 percent of all psychiatric beds to over 35 percent of nonfederal inpatient capacity today. As mentioned earlier, the proportion of psychiatrists who consider private psychiatric hospitals their primary place of employment has risen from 3 percent only 10 years earlier to more than 10 percent in 1988. Hospital growth in new geographic locations provides sites of work not previously available and expands access to psychiatric services, including specialty services such as treatment of children and adolescents, or substance abusers.

The breadth of psychiatric practice as reflected in subspecialization is impressive. Several new requests for recognition through specialty qualification of the ABPN have been introduced recently. In a field in which there is known to be significant unmet demand or need for services, there is also much latitude for segmentation. Whether the impact of these trends will be fragmentation of psychiatry or growth of the science and practice of the profession remains an issue for further investigation and discussion. What is clear is that psychiatry is fast becoming a house of many professions, each nearly as large as the whole of psychiatry itself fifty years ago. Psychiatrists now are involved significantly in administration and research, reflecting the diversification of the profession.

New patterns of professional activities are evolving in psychiatry, as in other medical specialties, as the profession adapts to rapidly changing socioeconomic and scientific influences. In the 1980s, these influences have included advances in treatments for major psychiatric disorders (e.g., new antipsychotic medications like Clozapine and new neuroradiologic diagnostic tests), new forms of economic pressures on practice, and a changing mix of characteristics of practitioners, work settings, training, and roles.

This brief presentation of information about the practice of psychiatry highlights a number of aspects of the changing patterns of practice in the profession that are consistent with our findings from studies of hospitals and community mental health centers. First, there is increasing involvement in private hospitals, the number of which, as we have seen earlier, has grown enormously during the past decade. In addition, psychiatrists continue to treat severely mentally ill patients, occupying among mental health practitioners the role of the medical specialist. As was the case for psychiatric hospitals, we see marked specialization among individual practitioners. Psychiatrists spend substantial amounts of time in non-paid work at community mental health centers, on average three to five hours per week. And consistent with the expansion over the past several years of organized specialty mental health settings—from roughly 3,000 in 1970 to more than twice that many today—there has been a tendency for psychiatrists to increase their participation in work in organizations, including hospitals, and to rely less on individual private practice. As a result, psychiatrists are increasingly influenced by the competitive pressures experienced by these provider organizations.

Purchase of Service Contracting

For over four decades, reform in American government has been driven in large part by a quest for greater accountability, intended to ensure that public dollars and government authority were not misused. The privatization of government services—services formerly supplied by the government and now contracted through private agencies—has often been advocated on the grounds that it enhances accountability in public spending (Linowes, et al., 1989; Savas, 1987; DeHoog, 1984). Yet, privatization represents a curiously paradoxical aspect of efforts to make government more accountable.

Contracting with private agencies is thought to discipline the performance of government-financed services by introducing market-based competition among providers. Yet these institutional arrangements may in fact weaken traditional methods for ensuring accountability in the public sector (Dorwart and Schlesinger, 1988; Schlesinger, et al., 1986). This can occur in a variety of ways. By increasing the number of providers and decentralizing administration, contracting can vastly complicate the efforts of state and federal legislators to oversee a program (Carter, 1983). By shifting the locus of service delivery to the private sector, contracting can attenuate legal requirements for due process that have been established for government-provided services (Schlesinger, et al., 1986). For example, when state governments directly provide services, they are legally accountable for the well-being of those using the facility, but if the state purchases these services, these same legal requirements do not always extend to the private agency providing care.

By shifting employment of service providers out of the public sector, the types of rewards and opportunities available to those providers also change. Providers employed directly by the public sector cannot profit from their activities in excess of salary. In contrast, those providing services under contract can often quite legally profit by their activities. This may create incentives to provide more services than needed (Schlesinger, et al., 1989), and may also attract a provider who is interested in maximizing short-run profits, rather than providing quality services over the long term (Dorwart and Schlesinger, 1988; Young, 1983; Shore and Levinson, 1983).

Contracting and CMHCs. To augment our earlier discussion of CMHCs, we wish to consider also the relationship of contracting and CMHCs. The Community Mental Health Act explicitly provided a limited amount of federal funds to CMHCs, with the expectation that they would seek other funding later from insurers or from local government. These resources were to be used, where necessary, to subsidize the care of those unable to pay for services.

Several factors led to a somewhat different evolution for CMHC funding, one that channeled far more state money than expected into the community mental health centers. As states began to develop more community-based programs during the 1970s, and put these out for bid, the CMHC in each community was often in the best position to win the contract. The Social Security Amendments of 1967 and 1974 had laid the groundwork for this development. This legislation allowed states to count donations to private agencies as part of their 25 percent requirement to match funding with federal contributions (Gilbert and Specht, 1979). With their substantial preestablished position in the community, CMHCs were typically far more able than newly established agencies to raise the resources for matching grants.

As private health insurers, particularly over the past decade, became more concerned with controlling their costs, the potential to cross-subsidize the care of the uninsured was greatly reduced from what had been expected. Thus, states concerned about mental illness among the uninsured were forced to channel increased resources to the CMHCs in order to maintain an adequate level of care for this population. As a result, states have become an important source of funding for CMHCs, and CMHCs have come to play an important role in many state mental health purchase-of-services-contracting (POSC) systems. In some states, their role is primarily one of direct service provider. In others, they serve more as fiscal intermediaries, taking state dollars and subcontracting to other agencies to provide services within their catchment areas. Under either of these circumstances, when mental health contracting is channeled primarily through CMHCs, notions of how best to pursue accountability will be shaped accordingly.

Competition and community mental health agencies. Data collected by us from 633 community mental health agencies (CMHAs) were analyzed (Clark and Dowart, 1992). CMHAs, which are largely providers of outpatient services, are playing an increasingly important role in treating those suffering from mental illness. According to NIMH sources, between 1969 and 1983 new admissions to all outpatient facilities increased by 133 percent while inpatient admissions rose only 27 percent (NIMH, 1990a). During approximately the same period, the number of organizations offering outpatient services grew by 32 percent. Mental health agencies, supported partly by governmental funds, are particularly important as a source of mental health care for low-income individuals; these agencies are often the only option available to those who are not insured or cannot pay the full price of treatment. CMHAs have also become important as a source of treatment for insurers and employers who have increasingly begun contracting with CMHAs to provide "managed care" to their employees.

Very little is known about how community mental health agencies respond to competition. While they are likely subject to many of the same pressures as are inpatient care facilities, it is plausible that they may respond differently because of the unique services they provide and the particular populations they serve. Analyses by us indicate that competition, as measured by the number of facilities per 100,000 population, has a clear impact on community mental health agencies. Interestingly, competition did not encourage more efficiency. Instead, higher levels of competition appeared to discourage group treatment and led agencies to be less concerned about maximizing client-derived revenues. Like hospital-based inpatient facilities, CMHAs under highly competitive conditions reduced the percentage of below-cost care provided.

Strategies or Responses to Competition

The market for health and mental health services is often characterized as monopolistically competitive; providers compete on the basis of price and quality (Klevorick and McGuire, 1987; Goldsmith, 1988). Many observers believe that quality-based competition has predominated over price competition, causing costs to rise in spite of increased competition. In mental health services, quality-based competition may take the form of specialization or, in economic terms, product differentiation. Thus, in an effort to create a perception of possessing special expertise, mental health providers may choose to focus on a particular form of mental health problem or population, e.g., eating disorders, child and adolescent disorders, substance abuse. From this perspective, as competition increases in a market area, more providers will attempt to carve out a niche by specializing. In more competitive market areas we would expect to find more specialists and, therefore, fewer generalists among mental health providers. In very competitive areas, where the market might more closely resemble perfect competition, it may become difficult for institutions to sustain a full array of traditional services. For example, an emergency service might not bring in a sufficient number of paying clients to be supportable under highly competitive conditions.

In sum, we distinguish between four competitive strategies that may be used by providers:

1. *Price competition* is characterized by practices that result in lower charges to consumers as compared to charges of other providers. These practices might include an emphasis on efficiency and the discouragement of treatment of costly patients, such as those with chronic illness or an inability to pay for treatment.

2. Providers competing on the basis of *quality* try to attract consumers by providing services and/or staff that are seen as better than that of competitors. This could be achieved, presumably, by providing special services or by hiring highly experienced or specially trained staff.

3. *Product differentiation* is an effort by a provider to set itself apart from other providers by focusing on a narrow spectrum of services and/or patients—for example, treatment of drug and alcohol dependence—thereby gaining a reputation for expertise in these areas.

4. In a fourth method, employing *oligopolistic strategies*, providers try to avoid direct competition through formal or informal agreements with potential competitors. Market competition is limited to competition among a small number of vertically integrated providers. For example, in an area where competition for inpatients is high among hospitals, one hospital may respond by expanding into outpatient services partly to establish a consistent source of referral. In response, individual provider groups already providing outpatient services, such as CMHAs, may try to establish exclusive arrangements with other hospitals.

EPILOGUE

In 1991, the newly elected Governor of Massachusetts, William Weld, announced that he would close several public hospitals (including three state mental hospitals) and consolidate their functions (Governor's Special

Commission, 1991). Necessary substitution services would be purchased through contracts with private general and specialty psychiatric hospitals (or nursing homes in the case of medical services for the elderly). This large-scale reform was just getting underway when this book was written. It does represent, however, one state government's prescription for the future direction of health and mental health care.

In a closely related move, the state announced that it would convert the Medicaid program for psychiatric and substance abuse services to a new, privately vendored, managed care system. A vendor has been selected to begin to set up a state-wide managed mental health care system for Medicaid recipients. It is anticipated that it will take one to two years before the new program is fully operational.

Both the consolidation of state facilities and the nascent managed care system have stirred debate, controversy, and opposition from advocacy and provider groups who argue that the benefits of privatization are unproven and that stringent management of care is unnecessary. This ambitious initiative is being viewed widely as an "experiment" whose outcome is uncertain. What is certain is that the changes will result in movement of services in the direction of private provision (although with public funding) and that there will be increasing emphasis on issues of management and accountability. We would expect similar changes to be proposed and implemented in many states. In both the next and in the last chapters of this book, we attempt to put into perspective our own analysis and findings and to suggest future directions for policymakers concerned with privatization in mental health.

Part III

PRIVATIZATION AND POLICIES FOR THE FUTURE

CHAPTER 7

Public-Private Partnerships: A Case Study of Cambridge, Massachusetts

This chapter consists of a "community case study" of the development of the mental health system in the City of Cambridge, Massachusetts. The first section describes the history and development of a "traditional" community mental health center in Cambridge. The next part describes the changes related to "privatization" from 1980 to 1990. The case study has two major themes. First, we demonstrate the evolution through the historical periods, described in Chapter 2, of mental health services in the context of one community. This is essentially the story of one community's experience in going from a situation where few mental health services existed to a comprehensive community mental health service system over a period of many years.

Second, we examine how more recently, during the 1980s, significant elements of the mental health system have moved in the direction of a privatized model of providing services that employ specialized and medicalized treatment models. These latter developments can be traced to the kinds of forces mentioned in the historical review in Chapter 2 and are illustrated also by national trends and by data from our surveys of psychiatric hospitals, community mental health centers and individual psychiatrist providers presented in Part Two of this book.

Our approach might be described as a "case within a case." First, we will discuss the program in the City of Cambridge and then we will turn to focus on the past decade at the Cambridge Hospital as it becomes a more central institution in the city's mental health programs and adapts to the pressures of privatization.

COLONIAL ERA, 1640–1800

Because there is relatively little documentation about health and mental health care in the colonial period specific to the City of Cambridge, we will briefly summarize here events in the Commonwealth of Massachusetts as well as those we know about the city. In 1641 the Bay Colony Body of Liberties included reference to allowances for "idiots and distracted persons," this language being similar to that used in England at that time. By 1645 the Governing Committee had to consider laws concerning "inmates, feeble-minded and aged persons." In 1676, there appeared the earliest legislation directly related to the care of the insane and giving authority to the selectmen of towns for their care. Later, in 1694, the jurisdiction for the care of the insane was delegated to the Overseers of the Poor. In 1730, we find the first mention of an insane person in the public records in the territory that is now called Cambridge. This case involves a man who was having so much trouble taking care of his son, who was psychotic, that he could not do his own work. The town agreed either to keep the son in jail at public expense or to require him to leave town. Much later, around 1784, the first guardianship laws of the commonwealth were drafted.

Increasing organization of the town government was evident by 1786 when the first Board of Overseers of the Poor for Cambridge was created. Specifically, the board had responsibility for the poorhouse and for accounting for the expenditure of tax funds in the care of indigent persons. At this time doctors to deliver personal health care were scant, and self-care and home remedies were the rule. There were no hospitals in Cambridge, private homes having been used to treat the injured during the Revolutionary War. In Boston, the practices of colonial times had begun to change, so that fewer itinerant surgeons and clergyman-doctors were practicing. While the forum of communal planning provided for some aspects of town development, health care was not among them. Neither public health regulation nor public medical services existed in Cambridge before 1800.

Although at that time there were no mental hospitals in Cambridge or elsewhere in Massachusetts, a poorhouse had been built in Cambridge in 1789. Residing in the poorhouse were indigent persons, some of whom would be identified today as mentally ill or retarded. Such persons were frightening and perceived as potentially dangerous; methods of constraint consisted of chains and cages. But some in the poorhouses were merely socially incompetent individuals, many of whom were immigrants. The homeless, family-less, the crippled, and the drunkard all populated the poorhouse, along with vagrants and common criminals. Indeed, it was this practice of mixing different groups of people that eventually led to the segregation of the mentally ill, especially the non-violent. This was done partly because caretakers believed the mentally ill should be separated because of their medical condition, as Pinel had argued successfully at the Salpetriere Hospital in Paris many years before (Zilboorg, 1941). Over-crowding and the resulting poor social conditions were the impetus for reformers to plead for segregation of the mentally ill and, soon, for the creation of separate private asylums modeled after the European retreats. One such was the McLean Hospital, which opened in what is now Somerville in the early nineteenth century (Sutton, 1986).

The early poorhouse reflected in its inception and functioning the dominant philosophy of that period. A series of poorhouses were con-structed in Cambridge, such as the one located on Prospect and Harvard streets and dedicated by Abiel Holmes, the prominent preacher and father of Dr. Oliver Wendell Holmes, Sr. We can learn something of the thinking of that early period by turning to the accounts written by Abiel Holmes.

At a special meeting of the Overseers of the Poor of the Town of Cambridge on September 17, 1818, the Reverend Doctor Holmes, then pastor of the First Church in Cambridge, delivered a "discourse" on the occasion of the opening of the new almshouse (Holmes, 1818). In Cam-bridge, the spirit of reform and charity was strong in the early nineteenth century, led by the religious leaders of the community. Holmes' remarks were about the poor, but they are also interesting if one considers them in the context of the legislation that led the overseers to establish the almshouse. He stressed that many kinds of people were among the poor, including many insane and retarded persons. The legislation clearly pro-vided for "commitment" to the almshouse of persons who were poor, indigent, refused or neglected to work, who engaged in "drinking, gaming, idleness and debauchery, and thereby involved themselves and their families in distress, misery and ruin," or who were imbeciles or handi-capped. The overseers saw their charge as that of providing "suitable support, tendance, and protection" for "the destitute, sick, and helpless."

In his discourse, Holmes set himself a task to consider the biblical assertion that "the poor will always be with us; the duty of relieving them, and the means by which we may do them the most good." Holmes was an articulate spokesman for the sentiments, beliefs, and, we would now say, *values* of this time. His observations are useful in at least three ways. First, he provides his own historical perspective. Second, he describes for us the conditions of the almshouse and its community setting. And third, he articulates the prevailing philosophy behind what would soon become a major public policy initiative, the asylum movement.

Holmes extols the wisdom and virtues of the current undertaking of the establishment of the almshouse by the City of Cambridge:

But although private charity can do much, public charity can do more; and though many of the poor always may and ought to be relieved by the one, it is the privilege of the most indigent classes of them, in all Christian countries, to have the benefit of the other. Such, eminently, is the privilege of the poor in our town, in our own Commonwealth. . . . In the observance of the law, this town has, I believe, been uniformly exemplary. . . . The house, in which we are convened . . . is large and well constructed. . . . Its apartments are well suited to the various ages and sexes, characters and conditions of those who may occupy them. . . . The sick will have suitable apartments assigned to them; be under the care of the attending physician; and have nurses appointed to take charge of them by night and by day, to see that their apartments are kept clean and all medications administered. . . . The present inhabitants of this asylum will greet you as their best friends and benefactors.

Holmes reveals some seeds of public charity that would grow over future years into a system of welfare programs, reform schools, hospitals, and insane asylums for providing services to a large proportion of people living in the city. Although he has no specific plan, he does have a philosophy. "In case of failure in an individual to perform them, where, but from the *community* can you expect a remedy? . . . Pain and want, although individual complaints, are actually sores upon the body politic; hence the necessity and the duty of the public to interfere for their relief."

It is interesting that nearly seventy years later, when the Cambridge physician and civic leader, Morrill Wyman, spoke at the dedication of the first Cambridge Hospital (now called the Mt. Auburn Hospital), he cast a skeptical if not critical glance at the now-outdated almshouse of Holmes' vision. In Wyman's words:

Although the sick in the almshouse are accommodated with a hospital room, and receive all the attention and kindly care possible under the circumstances, it is after all a poorhouse. It is a mingling of those who have become sick through no fault of their own, with the vicious, the degraded, those who have lost their citizenship and even the criminal. The surroundings of the sick, upon which so much depends, can be but slightly improved by gifts of money, the prescribed medications may not be got or, if got, not properly administered; nursing may be entirely wanting. Thus, money will be wasted and either the whole attempt fails for want of organization or becomes a most expensive, unsatisfactory form of charity. (Wyman, 1886)

Here we see the not very subtle change from the view that public charity could provide health care to the view that private institutional services were necessary—what Vogel has called "the invention of the modern hospital," which in fact was occurring about the time of the founding of this hospital in the late nineteenth century (Vogel, 1980).

CAMBRIDGE: NINETEENTH CENTURY

The Cambridge of 1800 was a relatively quiet place with a population of only a few thousand people. The revolutionary period was a generation past, and industrialization was not yet on the horizon. A village of about 200 homes clustered about a commons and a college, Cambridge depended on Boston for commerce, transportation, news, and fashion, and for medical advice and treatment. Politically, the commonwealth was free from British control, although strong economic ties remained. And in New England the principle of local control of town affairs by town government was strong. Social services remained largely non-governmental concerns, centered about the church, private philanthropy, and a few rudimentary government functions, such as police and jails, poorfarms and almshouses. A few unevenly trained private practitioners of medicine lived in the community at the turn of the century. Certain aspects of the city's future development were already evident: its early role as a seat of government in Massachusetts; its emergence as an intellectual center and its lifelong relationship with Harvard University; its rapid development in the nineteenth century from a rural village into an urban city; its evolution from separate geographic clusters, such as East Cambridge, Cambridgeport, and Old Cambridge, into a modern community of neighborhoods; and, perhaps most strikingly, its sociocultural diversity (Sutton, 1976).

The City of Cambridge, Massachusetts, was chartered in 1846. At about that time the stirrings of the first public health movement in Massachusetts were creating a ripple of public interest in such issues as clean water, sanitation, the control of infectious diseases, and the formation of governmental organizations to promulgate public health codes. Numerous social reformers, private charities, and prominent church leaders were bringing to the public's attention the plight of the infirm, disabled, feeble-minded, and insane persons. Six years before Cambridge was chartered as a city, Dorothea Dix visited a jail in East Cambridge, and began her crusade to establish more insane asylums. (See Chapter 2 and below.) Cambridge was fortunate to have among its citizens a number of men whose prominence as physicians and as public figures inspired its advances in public health. The Cambridge Board of Public Health was mandated in the first city charter, and counted among its members Henry P. Walcott, a physician who was one of the pioneers of public health activities in the United States. Earlier, the Cambridge physician Benjamin Waterhouse had brought attention to Cambridge through his appointment to the founding faculty of the Harvard Medical School, then located in Cambridge, and through his interest in smallpox inoculation.

It would be forty years after the ratification of the city charter before Cambridge opened its first general public hospital, the first Cambridge Hospital (now the Mt. Auburn Hospital), through the efforts of Walcott and Morrill Wyman, son of Rufus Wyman, the first Superintendent of McLean Asylum. The year 1886 also saw the opening of the Westborough State Hospital for the insane, where Cambridge's mentally ill or deficient residents were often sent, and creation of a State Board of Lunacy and Charity, separated from a newly created Board of Health. In 1909, the state officially assumed the financial responsibility from the towns for the care of the mentally ill and several more state hospitals were opened.

Dorothea Dix and Other Reformers

Dorothea Dix's first contact with the insane reportedly was in 1840 in the East Cambridge jail. Her plea to the state legislature is one of the most frequently cited documents in the history of mental health services and social policy in the state of Massachusetts, the "Memorial to the Legislature of Massachusetts" (Dix, 1843). This memorial is indeed a remarkable document inasmuch as it depicts, in graphic terms, the care of the insane in Massachusetts homes, houses and prisons around 1840. It is a powerful, passionate, and poignant testimonial, one that was to be repeated again and again by Dix in her role as a social reformer as she traveled throughout the United States, Canada, and Europe leading a crusade for the establishment of mental hospitals in the nineteenth century. After her emotional opening statement, Dix detailed in a series of lengthy vignettes and cases the stories of many unfortunate men and women residing in prisons and almshouses, describing their gradual deterioration of function over many years, their exposure to public ridicule, and the incompetent, neglectful and abusive treatment they received. She notes that "the greatest evils in regard to the insane and idiots in the prisons of this commonwealth are found at Ipswich and Cambridge, and distinguished these places only, as I believe, because the numbers were larger, being more than twenty in each."

In Chapter 2 we described how the nineteenth century was best known as the institutional period in the development of mental health care, and so it was in Cambridge as well. To illustrate the evolution of community mental health services, consider briefly the development of the Westborough State Hospital. The hospital is located on a piece of land that was granted to the second president of Harvard College, Reverend Chauncy, in lieu of salary for his services in 1659. Later, he sold the land to a private farmer in the town of Westborough, and eventually the town bought the land as a public holding. In the mid-nineteenth century the state of Massachusetts decided to establish the first reform school for so-called wayward youth, and they purchased the land surrounding the Chauncy Lake for this purpose. Buildings were constructed and the school opened in 1848. The Lyman Reform School developed over the next forty years into a remarkable institutional community for the education and reformation of these juvenile offenders, some of whom we would today consider to be mentally retarded or emotionally handicapped. The school had a working farm, an industrial workshop, a fully functional school and classrooms, and even a nautical division with seagoing ships anchored in New Bedford and Salem.

In the late nineteenth century, the "Homeopathic Medical Society" persuaded the legislature of the need for a state-supported hospital for the practice of homeopathic medicine and for a homeopathic insane asylum (Dorwart, 1989). The Lyman School site was chosen for use as a homeopathic asylum, and the school was relocated to new quarters nearby. The Westborough Asylum opened in 1886 modeled, like other nineteenth century state mental hospitals, on the moral treatment approach that was soon to decline in popularity. The homeopathic philosophy led to a variety of therapeutics employed at Westborough, including homeopathic doses of medicines and "rest therapy" (especially for women) as advocated by S. Weir Mitchell, a renowned Philadelphia physician interested in mental illness. As theories about biological influences on mental illness increased, the Westborough Hospital established a pathology laboratory under the direction of the noted black neuropsychiatrist, Solomon Carter Fuller. (Westborough State Hospital is located nearly forty miles from the City of Cambridge, and its location was to pose a problem for mental health planners in the community mental health center era in the 1960s; community programs were to be linked to state mental institutions, but were also expected to operate under the theory that treatment close to home was beneficial to patients.)

Social reformers like Horace Mann, Samuel Gridley Howe, and others made significant contributions during this time. The link to the earlier colonial period of nineteenth century American psychiatry and the later moral treatment movement has been remarked upon by Greenblatt: "Much that was embodied in moral treatment sprang from the warm regard of the early settler for his neighbor. It depended on small-group living, was nourished by close interpersonal contact, and included, by its very nature, a concern with continuity of care" (Greenblatt, 1984). The creation of community was an evolutionary process. We can take note of developments at this time both in the City of Cambridge and also in the state government's activities in organizing formal public health programs.

Cambridge as a City and a Community

By 1846 the city had distinctive zones of development, or neighborhoods, known as East Cambridge, Old Cambridge, and Cambridgeport. North Cambridge was developed later and was for a long time an agricultural area. East Cambridge was located in the area bounded by the Charles River on the east and Somerville on the north. Early bridges were built connecting Cambridge and Boston, and in the mid-1800s large numbers of immigrants, especially Irish, Italian, and Portuguese, moved into this area. There was much industrial development and, later, railroads were constructed. Today, immigration continues, with a sizable Portuguese population and small but growing Asian and Hispanic populations. Historically, development in East Cambridge has been related to the moving of the county courthouse for Middlesex County into that part of the city and also to industrialization. Industrialization brought numerous problems. For example, Millers River in East Cambridge became so polluted from waste from industries such as meat packing, glass, and soap factories that its condition became a major public issue in the mid-nineteenth century, leading to the creation of a state Department of Public Health to regulate sanitation and water supplies.

The idea that each community provided organized public services was well accepted in urban America in the mid-nineteenth century. By 1886, the year in which the Westborough State Hospital opened and the new Cambridge General Hospital treated its first patient, America according to Wiebel (1967) was in the throes of one of its recurrent crises of community identification. Confidence in the reigning mythology that expected each community to govern itself and care for its own people was crumbling under the weight of economic distress and technological progress. The reality, if not the ideal, of the island community was dissolving under the pressures of social change.

Public Health and the State

A shift from local responsibility to the involvement of the state in public health matters began officially in Massachusetts with the creation of a state Board of Health in 1869. As described by Gerald Grob (1973 and 1966), the state had already been providing mental health services for some forty years, following the establishment of the Worcester State Hospital. A pattern that saw developments in mental health services preceding those in the delivery of other public health and medical services recurred throughout the history of public health and mental health. According to Rosenkrantz (1972), the state Board of Health was established along the general principles that the state is responsible for controlling disease, and that its mission was to transfer moral and scientific knowledge into public policy. The first report of the Joint Special Commission to Consider the Expediency of Establishing a State Board of Health in Massachusetts in 1869 held forth the goal of a "healthy community" (Rosenkrantz 1972, p. 8).

Lemuel Shattuck was one of the early leaders of public health reform in Massachusetts. Shattuck considered himself a "statist," that is, a dealer in facts, and he was active in the American Statistical Association. But, perhaps equally important, he was a "statist" in another sense, that is, one who saw the responsibility of the state for providing for the public health. Shattuck pointed out in 1848 that the state of Massachusetts was already collecting sporadic statistics describing pauperism, crime, insanity, agriculture, banks, and insurance companies. A few years later, Dr. Edward Jarvis began the systematic collection of vital statistics on insanity on a statewide basis. Jarvis' report in 1855 on insanity and idiocy in Massachusetts proposed extending the state's responsibility to the institutional care of the insane. Coincidentally, Jarvis also practiced an unusual brand of community psychiatry in that he treated some insane patients in his home at that time.

The state Board of Health developed under the leadership of Dr. Henry Ingersoll Bowditch, and with the support within the medical community of his partner in practice, Dr. Morrill Wyman. Perhaps not surprisingly, given that the philosophy of the earlier colonial period was still in the minds of many, there was an emphasis among public health practitioners of the time on reforming individual character and behavior (Bockoven, 1972). For example, the state board assisted in the development of local Boards of Health and, as Rosenkrantz notes, "Freedom from disease was viewed as primarily a personal responsibility dependent upon the character and habits of the individual" (Rosenkrantz, 1972, p. 64). At the same time there was widespread acceptance of "moral treatment" in mental health. In 1886, the state Board of Health, Lunacy, and Charity was reorganized under the new state Board of Health, a separate and independent body that was chaired by Dr. Henry P. Walcott. As described by Rosenkrantz: "Moral behavior remained indispensable to the prevention of disease, but as sanitation and hygiene became more scientific, the privilege of establishing adequate standards of behavior became the prerogative of the knowledgeable and the possession of knowledge became the sanction of moral behavior" (p. 73). Thus, we might say that the principles of moral treatment had become institutionalized on a broad scale by the late nineteenth century. Individuals increasingly were expected to conform to the mores of the larger community and society, and when unable so to do, they were increasingly segregated and isolated.

Private Sector Programs in Historical Context

In Chapter 2 of this book we discussed a general history of services for the severely mentally ill. In this chapter, we review some history most relevant to this case study of privatization.

Few existing histories of mental health care in the United States fully address the different components of the mental health service system that include public state hospitals, general hospital psychiatric units, and private psychiatric hospitals (Gibson, 1978). The authors' current research attempts to examine simultaneously these different elements of the service system, and it is therefore appropriate for us to look at their history. As Brown (1985) has said, we need "a historically grounded political-economic approach that can describe the legacy of early asylum building and reform and articulate its present relationship to social, political, and fiscal forces" (p. 4). We must, in other words, look at historical context as well as at current policy to answer the question: What is the role of public and private resources in providing mental health services?

In the early nineteenth century, as more was learned about the classification and identification of individuals with mental illness, the value of treating mental illness in separate places was increasingly espoused: "However, it was found advisable by all those named that the wards for the insane should be separated from those appropriated to the ordinary sick and they are all now regarded an entirely different form of management. They have no connection with the parent institutions from which they originally sprung, except in being under the control of the same 'Board of Managers' " (Kirkbride, 1880 quoted in Vogel, 1980).

Although several private psychiatric hospitals had been opened in New England, non-affluent citizens still depended on the general hospitals, almshouses, and poorhouses for care. The same clamor from reformers for the separation of the mentally insane from the general sick that encouraged the birth of the private hospitals for the insane demanded that the state make some provisions for the indigent among them. We have described earlier the development of the state hospitals. In addition to state hospital care, some of the state's poor were treated in private hospitals under contract with the state, even in the early nineteenth century. In Massachusetts, Connecticut, and Vermont, as well as in other states that needed treatment for the quickly overflowing numbers of patients in the state institutions, contracting with private institutions took place. Tuke notes, "It is well known that in many states the contract for the care of the pauper insane, notably in New England, was awarded annually to the lowest bidder. This was not due to the fact that the insane were less considered than other dependents; it was the custom thus to make annual provisions for the care of paupers" (Tuke, 1813, p. 140).

In Connecticut, the Hartford Retreat, a private hospital established by the State Medical Society in 1824, cared for the insane under contract from the state during the period of forty years previous to the construction of state hospitals in Connecticut. The same is true of Butler Hospital at Providence, Rhode Island, which owed its establishment in 1847 to private benevolence and for many years cared for the insane who needed hospital care under contract with the state (Tuke, 1813). Although this early form of privatization was present at the inception of the state mental health systems, the extent of such contracting was limited. For example, the private hospitals were only under obligation to provide services for a specified number of days. From the mid-nineteenth century on, there developed on parallel but separate tracks the two sectors for psychiatric services, the public institutions and the private asylums. Little has been written about the private psychiatric hospital sector except for accounts of the individual private hospitals. These separate public and private sectors persisted well into the twentieth century and form the basis for our multi-tiered system of care.

General Hospital Psychiatry

Concurrently with the growth of psychiatry as a discipline came the increase in the importance of the role of the general hospital in mental health care. As mentioned earlier, psychiatric units in general hospitals in the United States date back to the nineteenth century at the Pennsylvania

Hospital and the Massachusetts General Hospital. Sederer et al. note, "Historically, the inpatient unit in the general hospital developed out of a need to relieve some of the burden of the public hospital as well as to provide local (community) psychiatric inpatient treatment in immediate proximity to where patients obtain their medical care" (1984). One reason general hospitals did not become the model for care of the mentally ill in the nineteenth century was that they were reluctant to care for the *indigent* insane. Because of reforms that made private and "public" (e.g., Medicare and Medicaid) insurance payments available to general hospitals for treating mentally ill patients who otherwise would not have been able to afford care, psychiatric care in general hospitals began to flourish and grew significantly in the middle of the twentieth century with the development of new medications that could treat serious mental illness. As health insurance became widely available, inpatient episodes in psychiatric units of general hospitals increased 25 percent between 1971 and 1981, according to Kiesler and Sibulkin (1987, p. 59).

With the growth of the general hospital inpatient unit, psychiatry as a profession also began to grow in prestige because the milieu of the general hospital offered psychiatrists legitimacy, education, and a network of colleagues in a way that the state mental hospital, or even perhaps private hospitals in an earlier time, could not. The general hospital psychiatric unit was considered a better environment for the patient because he or she could easily be treated for other medical problems in a diverse hospital, usually closer to home. General hospital psychiatrists would be significant later in staffing community health centers because of the flexibility allowed doctors in general hospitals who could have private practices in the community in addition to their responsibilities at the hospital. This dual practice was more difficult to arrange for professional employees of public mental hospitals.

Educators realized the training potential of the psychiatric unit in the general hospital and programs evolved for psychiatric residents and other trainees. Today the public general hospitals have the highest proportion of psychiatric trainees per hospital of any type of institution. This training function began as early as 1900 when, for example, the New York Hospital in Albany opened a psychiatric ward, citing their goals as the following: "(1) Care for acute mental illness; (2) standards of care equal to those applicable in general medical wards; (3) treatment close to the community without the stigma of mental hospitalization; and (4) *training for interns and residents*" (Barton, 1986, p. 151).

With the growth of psychiatry as a profession, the state hospitals became but one setting for practice by emerging students of psychiatry as they began to find success at private practice and in general hospitals.

With the increasing numbers of teaching and clinical positions becoming available in University medical centers, and the parallel growth in the intellectual relevance of dynamic views, the state hospitals grew progressively less attractive to many able and well educated young psychiatrists. (Kriegman et al., 1975, pp. 141–42)

COMMUNITY MENTAL HEALTH CENTER MOVEMENT

The modern community mental health center is an example of a bridging or transitional institution linking previously separate institutions, the state mental hospitals and the community general hospitals. Superficially, the community mental health center movement represented a reorganization of mental health services in the United States to emphasize outpatient treatment over state hospital care. Were this all that community mental health represented, there would be relatively little controversy surrounding its public policy implications, little doubt about its success in shifting of emphasis at national, state, and local levels, and little interest in examining its history. But the community mental health movement took on the proportions of a social movement involving medicine, public health, and social welfare institutions, and it stirred controversy across the country. This seemingly benign philosophy of providing more outpatient mental health services came to symbolize the struggle for improved human services and mobilized both support and, at times, opposition from professional, political, ethnic, civil rights, and community constituencies.

Changes after World War II

Grob (1987) has described the dramatic changes that have taken place over the past forty years in psychiatry and in community mental health programs in the United States. One way to look at these changes is to compare the services that were available then and now. We will briefly sketch this comparison for the United States as a whole and then return to the history of change in the City of Cambridge.

Immediately after World War II, the Group for the Advancement of Psychiatry was formed (Grob, 1987). This group of psychiatrists was concerned with the general status of organized psychiatry in America and undertook to write a series of reports to inform the profession and the general public (GAP, 1948, 1949). One of their early reports dealt with the status of services. In 1948 most care was provided in poorly staffed public hospitals. At that time, most funds for mental health services came from public (state) sources and went to government-operated institutions; roughly 95 percent of psychiatric hospital patients were in government institutions. Today most psychiatric patients are either treated in private hospitals or in nongovernmental outpatient clinics and community mental health centers. Moreover, more than half of direct care expenditures are obtained from third-party payments (including Medicaid, Medicare, and Social Security Disability Insurance (SSDI) (McGuire, 1989a). At mid-century there were 4,000 psychiatrists, 2 percent of all physicians; today there are roughly 35,000 psychiatrists, or 6 percent of all physicians. Then there were 150 psychiatric units in general hospitals; today there are ten times that number. Reportedly, hospital staffing ratios and minimum "standards" of the American Psychiatric Association were appallingly low in comparison to today's conditions: one psychiatrist per 200 patients, one social worker per 100 patients, one psychiatric nurse per 30 patients. By comparison, today we consider that a general hospital psychiatric unit should have a nurse-to-patient ratio of one to two to be acceptable and one to one as optimal (NIMH, 1984). There were at that time 850 mental health clinics, 90 percent under public auspices. In 1990, in contrast, there were 1,500 community mental health centers, 1,200 day treatment programs, and 1,200 community residences (NIMH, 1990a). Thus there has been an enormous expansion of mental health services in the United States in the last forty years, and this growth and diversification is expected to continue (Thompson, 1982; NIMH, 1990a).

MENTAL HEALTH SERVICES IN CAMBRIDGE SINCE WORLD WAR I

The lull in progress in the United States in psychiatric care of the mentally ill early in this century, described earlier, was evident as well in Cambridge. Sigmund Freud's ideas were emerging but were not yet thought to be useful in treating the seriously mentally ill. Following World War I, however, a series of important institutional events marked the emergence of what was to become the community mental health movement in Massachusetts and the basis of the Cambridge-Somerville community mental health center. In 1917 the Cambridge City Hospital (now called the Cambridge Hospital) was founded to serve the medically indigent of the community. Soon afterward the Massachusetts Division of

Mental Diseases was established. By this time, the beginnings of the mental hygiene movement were taking shape. (See Chapter 2.)

The last of the traditional state mental hospitals in Massachusetts was completed in 1933, the Metropolitan State Hospital in Waltham. The Department of Mental Health was officially created shortly thereafter, in 1938. Progress toward community mental health services in Cambridge was slow during the Depression and World War II. An outpatient clinic of Westborough State Hospital began at the Mt. Auburn General Hospital in 1947, followed by the founding of the Cambridge Child Guidance Clinic in 1955, and by a day-care center in 1962.

In 1955 there were few organized mental health services in the City of Cambridge. The Child Guidance Clinic had just been founded, with one psychiatrist, one social worker, a nurse, and a secretary as the professional staff provided by the Department of Mental Health under the partnership clinic model. The clinic was sponsored by the Mental Health Association in Cambridge. Neither the Mt. Auburn General Hospital nor the Cambridge City Hospital had psychiatric units at that time. Some community agencies and church-sponsored social service organizations, such as the Catholic Charities, offered counseling. The state hospital used by Cambridge residents needing long-term care was located in Westborough, Massachusetts, nearly forty miles away; some mentally ill residents of the city who were expected to respond to short-term therapy were treated at the Massachusetts Mental Health Center in Boston or the Danvers State Hospital. In addition, private facilities such as McLean Hospital were used by those who could pay for their care. There were very few private practitioners of psychiatry at that time, although several psychoanalysts had offices located in Cambridge; there were no psychiatric services available in the nearby City of Somerville.

By the 1980s the situation had changed dramatically. The Cambridge-Somerville Mental Health Center and its affiliated programs had an operating budget of more than $5 million. There were more than fifty different programs or operating units within the mental health system in the city and over 500 staff involved in the care of patients. A general psychiatry residency training program served some twenty-five full-time psychiatrists in training. There were, in fact, not only all of the basic required elements of a comprehensive community mental health center in place: inpatient, outpatient, day treatment, emergency services, and community education and consultation programs, but many other services as well. Specialized programs existed for individuals with substance abuse disorders, mental retardation, emotional disorders of childhood, and dementia in the elderly, to name but a few.

Stages of Development in the Cambridge Hospital

Over the past twenty-five years there has been remarkable growth and change at the Cambridge Hospital and especially in its Department of Psychiatry. From 1965 to 1990, the hospital's budget increased fivefold (from roughly $10 million to $50 million annually) and the Department of Psychiatry was larger in 1990 (in terms of budget, staff, and training programs) than was the entire hospital in 1965. By 1990, the hospital and mental health center that were founded as "public institutions" had evolved and undergone a transformation. In 1991, the hospital was beginning construction of an "ambulatory care center" that was as large as the hospital itself, and the Department of Psychiatry had been "privatized" so that none of its more than 100 former state employees worked for the common-wealth. By examining this growth and transformation from a small municipal hospital to a widely recognized health and mental health center, we can learn a great deal about the evolution of care from hospitals to communities and from public provision to private models of service delivery.

Significantly, the Cambridge Hospital Department of Psychiatry was founded in 1965 shortly after passage of the landmark federal Community Mental Health Act and one year after the Massachusetts Community Mental Health Act was passed. Originally an outgrowth of the well-known and long-established training program of the Harvard Medical School at the Massachusetts Mental Health Center, the Cambridge program was from the outset designed to be part of a comprehensive community mental health and retardation center. Once the mental health center and its academically-affiliated Department of Psychiatry were joined, they grew together—merging one organization based in the community and its service programs with another based in a teaching hospital and its training programs. The services were upgraded, expanded, and changed; the training was broadened, enlarged, and modified. A new training orientation known as psychodynamic community psychiatry emerged in a relatively short time; the hospital organized a training program and defined new roles for psychiatrists working in the public sector. Together with training in community medicine, primary care, and neighborhood public health, psychiatric training at Cambridge Hospital evolved beyond the theories and practice common in 1965 to constitute a new form of social psychiatry.

The CMHC Movement, Beginnings in Cambridge

In 1964 at the age of fifty the Cambridge Hospital was reborn. On October 1, 1914, the mayor of Cambridge had appropriated funds previously authorized by the voters and the City Council and "thereupon the Trustees undertook the work" (City of Cambridge, 1917). But their hope of realizing the Progressive Era's reformist impulses had failed to thrive; the hospital had in fact become an embarrassment for the city in the 1960s when President Johnson's Great Society aspirations saw "bold new approaches" appropriate for community health and mental health programs. Following a scorching exposé of the hospital in a 1961 NBC white paper, a second-generation institution was proposed and a new hospital conceived. The City of Cambridge would erect a new hospital building and Harvard University would engage in an academic affiliation with the hospital. The match was publicly announced on June 24, 1965.

Clearly the rebirth of the hospital was more than material; it was also to be an intellectual and psychological rediscovery of institutional identity, analogous to what William James described for individual personalities as twice-born. The elements of the new institutional identity would be the established sense of community in Cambridge (Sutton, 1976), a major, ongoing commitment of time and effort by the university, and personal leadership from individuals who would continue the work begun by the first trustees fifty years earlier. All of these elements and more would be needed for success. Derek Bok, then President of Harvard University, wrote of this mid-1960s period: "In a disturbing number of cases, projects undertaken with high hopes met with failures that actually heightened local suspicions and frustrations rather than improving relations with the university" (Bok, 1982).

Cambridge City Hospital had opened to patients in 1917, three years after funding by the mayor of the proposal for Cambridge to have its "own hospital." There were not then or for some time to come psychiatric wards in most general hospitals and the "noisome patients" (City of Cambridge, 1917) at the Cambridge Hospital would, if they were determined to be insane and in need of public services, be sent to the designated district mental hospital at Westborough. Thus the hospital grew typically without a psychiatric service; it was not until the hospital's rebirth 50 years later that a Department of Psychiatry was established.

In the 1960s, the discipline of psychiatry itself was in the midst of an identity crisis, struggling to integrate the reawakening of its ties to medicine, its rediscovery of the community as a natural treatment setting, and in Cambridge as elsewhere, its emergence as a profession with a role in the life of a teaching hospital. At Harvard, an "Ad Hoc Committee Appointed to Consider How Best to Strengthen Psychiatry at Harvard" convened to review policies in light of the emergence of general hospital psychiatry services elsewhere. Although there were numerous psychiatric services affiliated with the medical school, the committee elected to focus on the teaching and research role of the Massachusetts Mental Health Center located adjacent to the Medical School, under the direction of the former Massachusetts Commissioner of Mental Health, Dr. Jack Ewalt.

Dr. John E. Mack, a psychiatrist at the Massachusetts Mental Health Center, was appointed Junior Visiting Physician in Psychiatry at the Cambridge Hospital on March 18, 1966. His appointment was officially in the Department of Medicine because there was then no Department of Psychiatry. He had been intrigued by the possibilities for breaking new ground at Cambridge in 1964 when he heard about plans for an academic affiliation between the Harvard teaching service at the Boston City Hospital and the Cambridge City Hospital. The affiliation would include a psychiatric service in Cambridge and Dr. Mack was excited about the proposed program because it would launch psychiatric services as an important participant in community medicine. This was virgin territory, for there existed in Cambridge at that time, as was common in other towns in Massachusetts, only a few community services: the Child Guidance Clinic, a day treatment program located at Fresh Pond, and as a resource, the state hospital in Westborough.

Dr. Mack was encouraged by Dr. Ewalt to explore the possibilities at Cambridge City Hospital for several reasons. Because of his familiarity with mental health services statewide from his tenure as Commissioner of Mental Health in Massachusetts, Dr. Ewalt knew there was a shortage of adult psychiatric services in the City of Cambridge. Introducing psychiatry at Cambridge would not only help the hospital, but the opportunity for medical consultations would be useful as a training experience for psychiatric residents at the Massachusetts Mental Health Center, a specialty psychiatric hospital. Dr. Ewalt thought that the Child Guidance Clinic already established in Cambridge would be an asset to Dr. Mack's program since it had ties to the Massachusetts Mental Health Center through its director, Dr. Robert Reid. Moreover, it was apparent in 1965 that federal grants would soon be available for the development of community mental health centers, especially in the areas where none currently existed. Members of the Cambridge Mental Health Association and Dr. Dana Farnsworth of the Harvard University Health Service in Cambridge were planning to apply for a federal mental health center grant. Several lines of development were thus coming together simultaneously at the beginning of 1965: the affiliation of Cambridge City Hospital with Harvard Medical School, the receptivity of the hospital to having a psychiatrist work with the Department of Medicine, and the interest of the medical school in developing psychiatric training programs.

A major change took place in Cambridge with the establishment in 1968 of a federally-funded (with matching state support) community mental health center. This single event, more than any other, accounted for the development of mental health services in the City of Cambridge in the next twenty-five years. In order to obtain a federal grant, an agency planning a community mental health center had to be prepared to offer inpatient, outpatient, and emergency services. Consequently, the Cambridge Mental Health Association, which hoped to found a CMHC, turned to the Cambridge City Hospital for a partnership in providing the required services. The Cambridge Hospital at that time was a municipal hospital that was by all reports in poor condition, with a reputation for inadequate medical services. The medical school would provide faculty to supervise hospital medical services in return for making the Cambridge Hospital one of its teaching hospitals for medical students. The city also decided to build a new hospital. As part of the overall affiliation agreement, the Massachusetts Mental Health Center, located in Boston, agreed to send staff psychiatrists to Cambridge City Hospital to consult on psychiatric cases.

Dr. John Mack and several others began these consultations in 1965 and 1966, thus laying the groundwork for the establishment of a Division of Psychiatry within the Department of Medicine at the hospital in 1967; later, when the CMHC proposal was funded, they established a Department of Psychiatry in the Cambridge Hospital to provide inpatient, outpatient, and emergency services. Other psychiatrists were recruited to work in the programs, which grew rapidly between 1968 and 1970. The roughly $1 million federal grant for the CMHC was accompanied, as required by law, by a commitment from the state Department of Mental Health to continue the funding for the center programs and staff after federal funding was phased out.

In the late 1960s, with help from faculty members from Harvard Medical School and Harvard Public Health School, a city-wide health department and a comprehensive system of health services, including neighborhood health centers, were established in the neighborhoods described earlier in this chapter. The Department of Psychiatry also became involved in this service delivery system, described by Macht et al. (1977) in *Neighborhood Psychiatry*. Numerous other specialty programs, for example, in drug abuse and alcoholism services, were being set up at this time. In addition, a National Institute of Mental Health funded residency training grant was obtained, and psychiatric residents began to work for the first time in 1972. Expanded collaboration occurred between the city and the state programs, not only in providing training services, but also in an increased affiliation with Westborough State Hospital and the development of community aftercare services. The training program reflected an active community psychiatry orientation combined with more traditional psychodynamic psychotherapy education. These programs continued to expand and evolve to create an academic mental health center up until 1980. After that time, the mental health center was almost wholly without federal funding and, like other community mental health centers in the post-1980 period, had to begin planning for its own fiscal self-sufficiency.

Mental Health Services in Cambridge and Privatization

One advantage in examining the development of mental health services in a single community is that linkages among general medical, mental health, and social service systems can be clearly identified and documented. Cambridge provides a good illustration of the local involvement and social activism characteristic of the 1960s and 1970s in developing mental health services. The city obtained the first federally-funded community mental health center in Massachusetts, which became a good example of a particular model of a center, namely, one based in a general hospital. The strong affiliation with Harvard Medical School was an unusual ingredient in the growth and development of the center. In the 1980s, this center and its affiliated Department of Psychiatry began an extensive process of "privatization" away from the purely public model of a community mental health center, providing an example of a development increasingly common. A description of how this hybrid public-private model for providing mental health services came about is the subject of the next part of this case study.

To illustrate how privatization has influenced the delivery of community mental health services, we describe next the experience of the Cambridge-Somerville Mental Health Center based at the Cambridge Hospital in Massachusetts in the decade 1981–1991. It is first useful briefly to review the federal and state background events in Cambridge.

During the 1980s the privatization of governmental services occurred generally throughout the United States. The policies of newly-elected President Ronald Reagan emphasized deregulation, degovernmentalization, and a "new federalism" that resulted in ceding back to state governments many responsibilities for social programs that had been carried out nationally. This trend also affected mental health policy and programs. Under President Jimmy Carter, the federal government had developed plans for expansion of the CMHCs that were created by Congress as the Mental Health Systems Act of 1980. This legislation was promptly repealed after the election of 1980 and replaced by a new and more comprehensive (but less generously funded) block grant to the states for alcohol, drug abuse, and mental health services. During the 1980s the trend of states purchasing services from private providers, including health and mental health services, fueled continued expansion of private providers and cutbacks in state-owned services (Davidson, et al., 1991).

The practice of contracting for mental health services grew in Massachusetts as well; by 1987 more than 50 percent of all state mental health services and 90 percent of all drug abuse services (funded through the Department of Public Health) were privately provided (Schlesinger, et al., 1986). This pattern of privatization was evolving in concert with continued efforts at "deinstitutionalization," which sought to move patient care from long-term inpatient care facilities into community-based residences, partial hospitalization programs, and outpatient clinics. Contracting for services, which was intended to foster competition, also gave rise to some large vendor-agencies. Established CMHCs, hospitals, or human service organizations were well positioned to grow and diversify as they competed to provide local services. In Cambridge, the Department of Psychiatry at the Cambridge (municipal) hospital was one such institution that participated in this new entrepreneurial approach to providing mental health services.

By 1980, the Department of Psychiatry at the Cambridge Hospital was largely without federal funding for community mental health services because of the planned phasing out of federal subsidies. Achieving fiscal self-sufficiency was a difficult transition from the earlier phase of community and neighborhood psychiatry programs funded by federal and state grants. The then chief of psychiatry (Lee Macht, M.D.) died suddenly and was replaced by a new chairman (Myron Belfer, M.D.) who would direct the programs from 1981 to 1991. During this decade several initiatives were undertaken that involved shifts in funding of programs, new organizational affiliations, development of subspecialty programs, emphasis on research in addition to teaching, and entrepreneurial ventures. This process of diversification and differentiation resulted in growth of the institution and its role in the community and in the academic life of the university; however, it also resulted in the gradual transformation of the mental health programs. These transformations have influenced important aspects of mental health policy, such as who is treated, how and where they are treated, who pays for services, and the organization and governance of local mental health centers.

Deinstitutionalization

Deinstitutionalization is a philosophy that has influenced mental health policy in the United States for over thirty years (see our discussion in Chapter 2). As we trace the progress of deinstitutionalization in Cambridge, we begin to see how this major trend intersects with more recent policies of privatization. In the mid-1960s nearly all public inpatient psychiatric care was provided at a district state mental hospital (then Westborough State Hospital) that served people living in Cambridge. In the early 1970s the Department of Psychiatry at Cambridge Hospital established an affiliation for residency training at Westborough and through the Cambridge-Somerville Mental Health Center became increasingly involved in providing community services to former hospitalized patients. The growth of inpatient services especially reflects the tendency toward privatization of services from then (1960s) until the present and we will briefly recount these events.

In 1968, a twenty-bed psychiatric unit was established at the Cambridge Hospital which served a wide mix of patients (Cotton, et al., 1979). Because it was a municipal hospital, patients who were uninsured and who lived in Cambridge could be treated on this unit; since it was also a general hospital unit, patients with Medicaid, Medicare, and other insurance reimbursement were eligible for treatment. In the early 1970s, professional staff from Cambridge Hospital increasingly worked at the state hospital, where at about this time the census began to decline from the over 200 patients on the wards designated for Cambridge and Somerville residents (Dorwart, 1988).

A number of subsequent developments reflect the gradual and far-reaching movement toward further deinstitutionalization from the state hospital and toward privatization of mental health services. General hospital psychiatric units were opened at the private Mt. Auburn Hospital in Cambridge (sixteen beds) and at Central Hospital, a nonprofit hospital in Somerville with twenty beds initially and later thirty beds (twenty for involuntary patients). (In the mid-1980s, Central Hospital was purchased and continues to operate as a for-profit hospital as part of a multihospital corporation.) The number of community residences (or halfway houses) in the community increased from 10 in 1980 to 100 in 1990 to 150 in 1992. At the same time, the census at the Westborough State Hospital gradually declined to fewer than 100 patients in 1983, at which time the remaining patients were moved to Metropolitan State Hospital. In 1985, Cambridge Hospital bid for and received a contract from the state mental health authority to provide professional services at Metropolitan State Hospital.

By 1991, this state hospital had only fifty patients. In 1992, the state hospital was closed and the remaining patients moved to Cambridge or dispersed throughout the state.

In 1990 the state Department of Mental Health announced a reorganization, consolidation, and further privatization of mental health services. After Metropolitan was closed, Cambridge Hospital added twenty beds to accommodate some of those patients formerly in the state hospital; community-residential service agencies treat the others and have substantially replaced state hospital services. Only long-term care for uninsured patients remains the exclusive function of the state Department of Mental Health, and in 1991 the state expressed a willingness to contract with private specialty psychiatric hospitals to provide care on a per-diem basis for some of the patients in the four remaining state facilities. Over the past thirty years the census in these Massachusetts state mental hospitals has declined from over 20,000 to approximately 1,000 persons.

Cambridge Hospital Department of Psychiatry—Organization

Another unusual aspect of this case study is the role of the educational function and the university in the development of local mental health programs. The organizational and educational context of the Cambridge Hospital Department of Psychiatry is important. The Cambridge Hospital is a 200-bed, community general hospital. The major academic affiliation for the hospital is with the Harvard Medical School and this is true for the department of psychiatry as well. Among the many hospitals affiliated with Harvard Medical School, the Cambridge Hospital is perhaps best known for its training in community medicine and primary care, and among the departments of psychiatry at Harvard, the Cambridge program places relatively greater emphasis on training in community psychiatry. The residency training program, begun in 1972, now has forty residents and fellows in training in the adult psychiatry program, and eight residents in child psychiatry fellowship training. To summarize, the residency training program is based in a community general hospital with major affiliations with a CMHC, as well as with a university academic department. To date, more than 100 psychiatric residents have completed training at Cambridge Hospital.

Besides the intellectual environment provided by a formal training program, there is an impetus toward staying up-to-date that accompanies most training programs: guest speakers and consultants visit regularly, expectations for learning the latest innovations in treatment are high, accreditation requirements must be maintained. Training must also be relevant to the needs of the trainees and also to some extent to the changing professional marketplace. In psychiatry, more than 50 percent of individuals entering residency training in 1990 are women and this was also true at Cambridge Hospital. Increasing numbers of newly trained psychiatrists are taking positions in private hospitals and fewer are entering solo private practice; this trend also is evident in Cambridge. Thus, there is a tendency for developments in the field (such as privatization) to influence training through a subtle "feedback loop" wherein trainees must be prepared for their future careers.

Contracting for Services

As mentioned earlier, one of the major ways in which mental health services are provided in Massachusetts is through contracts from the state government. In Cambridge, a number of contracts were received by the Department of Psychiatry or affiliated organizations. One of the major affiliated organizations was the North Charles Foundation for Mental Health, Research, and Education. This foundation received contracts and then employed providers from the hospital to provide particular services specified by the state. Eventually many of these contracts were transferred to the hospital itself. For example, psychiatric residency training programs are provided through a contract with the state Department of Mental Health.

Many smaller contracts for providing aftercare services, day treatment programs, case management, and drug abuse treatment services were negotiated using a variety of reimbursement and accounting mechanisms. The organization, whether it be the foundation or the hospital, could more effectively blend funding from a variety of resources in order to create program budgets. To illustrate, a day treatment program might receive a contract from the state, insurance funds from private payers (e.g., Blue Cross/Blue Shield), and Medicaid or Medicare for eligible recipients from SSDI. Additional contracts for the day treatment program might come from a vocational rehabilitation agency, the Department of Public Welfare, or local HMOs. Of course, some patients also pay all or part of their fees from private or personal resources.

Specialization

The trend toward subspecialization in psychiatry has been widely recognized for many years. In medicine there are more "specialists" than primary care or family practitioners. In psychiatry there are now over thirty-five subspecialties, many of which are recognized by special board certification or similar recognition, such as child psychiatry, forensic psychiatry, geriatric psychiatry, substance abuse treatment, psychopharmacology, and so forth (Dorwart, et al., 1992a). This specialization has been driven by a number of factors such as advances in the science and therapeutics underlying treatment of different disorders that called for further training of care givers, the professional interests of providers, the recognized special needs of various subpopulations, and often, the structure of financial incentives in the medical profession. Similarly, among organizations, pressures towards diversification of services occurred as a response toward competition and as a means for expansion. This has been noted in CMHCs (Clark and Dorwart, 1992) and for psychiatric hospitals (Dorwart, et al., 1992b; Dorwart and Epstein, 1991). The Department of Psychiatry at Cambridge Hospital had a well-established, comprehensive service program and it was well positioned to begin further expansion, growth, and diversification. One of the ways in which this was accomplished was through the development of specialty services.

One of the first areas to be developed was child psychiatry. A child psychiatry residency (or fellowship) program had operated in the department for many years but there were no inpatient or outpatient services provided at the hospital. Therefore, a planning process was begun in 1981 which resulted in an approval for a certificate of need to construct a new psychiatric inpatient ward for children; this was completed and opened in 1990. In 1991, the development of an outpatient child psychiatric clinic was being actively pursued. The child training program has been expanded and a number of other specialty services were being provided, such as consultation to the schools and other community agencies.

A specialty treatment program established early in the history of the department was one geared to drug abuse and alcoholism treatment. Over time and especially in the late 1980s the program expanded to include a range of services such as methadone maintenance programs for heroin addiction, programs for individuals addicted to cocaine, and inpatient detoxification for drug and alcohol abusers.

A "victims of violence" program had its roots in programs concerned with the prevention of and treatment for rape, incest, and other sexual abuse. The program has expanded and grown rapidly to address other kinds of post-traumatic conditions related to war, community disasters, and the like. Each of these programs described in this section not only developed a discrete set of clinical services, but also its own array of educational and research programs.

Other types of specialty services actually may be viewed as generic services that cut across the other traditional and newer specialty services. For example, support for families with a member who has a major psychiatric disorder, and treatment of troubled couples and families with disturbed children all have been developed. A group therapy program to treat patients for a wide variety of disorders was established. A "psycho-pharmacology" clinic was founded in the mid-1980s and grew rapidly to provide consultation not only to the other clinical services, both inpatient and outpatient, but also to provide primary treatment services to large numbers of patients for somatic therapies where appropriate. As with the other services mentioned in this section, the psychopharmacology services could be reimbursed by public and private insurance. Patients were drawn to receive these services not only from the local community or "catchment area," but also from throughout Boston. Specialty services thus created a network of referral services for the hospital, another manifestation of privatization.

Another variation on specialization was the establishment of clinics to treat targeted populations of Portuguese, Latino, Haitian, and other minority populations needing translation services and ethnic sensitivities. Each of these programs developed its own leadership, staff, locations, and identity within the contexts of the CMHC and the hospital. As with other programs mentioned in this section, these programs received diversified funding, including contracts from the state department of mental health, other grants from federal and state government, and reimbursement from Medicaid, Medicare, and other insurers.

A range of other specialized services also developed over time, which cannot be described in detail; geriatric services, emergency services including a mobile crisis intervention team, outreach services to the homeless, case management services, and so forth. The description of these specialty services provides a picture of the way in which an organization can grow even when categorical resources are constrained, by diversifying and attracting patients from beyond the local area who have a variety of insurance mechanisms for paying for services received.

Organizational Affiliations

One of the ways in which the traditional public mental health center extended itself organizationally to become a more privately-oriented institution was through a network of affiliations and organizational arrangements. Often these affiliations were related to academic projects or training programs; however, in some instances they involved entirely new and innovative initiatives. Examples of Cambridge academic affiliations included a residency training program with the nearby HMO, the Harvard Community Health Plan. Another similar arrangement was with the New England Memorial Hospital, a private, not-for-profit, religiously-affiliated hospital, that provided training on a children's inpatient ward for the child psychiatry fellows. Similarly, affiliations were formed with the nearby Mt. Auburn Hospital for internship and residency training, and with Austen-Riggs Hospital in Stockbridge, Massachusetts for advanced residency training. In each instance the host institution provided a stipend for the trainee and also provided supervision from its faculty for the training program. Many other examples could be cited of exchanges between the Cambridge Hospital and other private institutions.

Organizational Diversification

Another initiative of the department of psychiatry was the creation of a proprietary subsidiary for providing supplemental psychiatric services to other hospitals. This venture was called the Cambridge Psychiatric Associates (CPA), which provided consultation or psychiatric services to a wide range of hospitals throughout greater Boston and to a few hospitals in other parts of New England. The privately-held entity developed contracts with private hospitals that paid for the services provided by individual psychiatrists at various community hospitals. A management function was also provided by CPA. At various times, CPA also developed outpatient clinics, consultation programs to schools, educational conferences, professional recruitment and placement services, and the like. In order to carry out these services, it was necessary for CPA to develop its own capacity through a subcontract for management functions at the North Charles Foundation to provide its own billing services, and its own physician practice group. The innovativeness of this arrangement is not in the activities themselves, which are quite common, but in the fact that a public hospital and mental health center had developed such an organization along a private corporate model with the explicit intent of providing subsidies for the ongoing core programs of the department and its staff.

Academic Programs

During the 1970s, a psychiatric residency training program had been established in the Department of Psychiatry at Cambridge Hospital, which is affiliated with Harvard Medical School. Over time the program grew and attracted physicians seeking training in clinical psychiatry. During the

1980s academic programs expanded markedly with increasing emphasis on sponsored research, continuing medical education for programs, advanced and specialized residency training (for example, child psychiatry or research), and expansion of efforts in medical student education and a host of other more specialized scholarly ventures involving institutes, centers, or consortia for the pursuit of the study of specific problems. For example, the Erikson Center was established to study the psychosocial factors related to individual and social development, and a Harvard Center for Addiction Studies and the Center for Studies in the Nuclear Age were established at the Cambridge Hospital, to mention only a few.

As a deliberate strategy, the department established relationships with departments and divisions of nearby Harvard University. In particular, education and research efforts were established between the Department of Psychiatry and the Department of Social Medicine at the medical school, and with the School of Public Health, the John F. Kennedy School of Government, the Graduate School of Education and the Departments of Psychology and Sociology in the Harvard College of Arts and Sciences. These programs grew in importance and scope and have provided an intellectual network and a sense of scholarly community for the department. In this way, the formal affiliation with Harvard Medical School not only was useful to the establishment of formal training programs in specific disciplines, but also the proximity and the interconnections with a university provided a strong intellectual basis for the growth and support of the individual faculty members, fellows, and students. Ties were also formed with a variety of other professional schools for social work, nursing, and psychology in the greater Boston area. We will briefly review a specific example of these education programs to illustrate the privatization of the formerly primarily public academic mental health center.

Continuing Medical Education

One of the many programs developed in the department of psychiatry was the continuing medical education (CME) conference series. This initiative was begun in the mid-1970s as an outgrowth of smaller intradepartmental educational lecture series and conferences. Over a fifteen-year period the conference series grew from small two- or four-hour sessions involving 50 to 100 people to half a dozen or more large annual conferences with 500 to 1,000 participants. Initially the topics of these conferences were oriented toward clinical practice and were related to basic issues such as psychotherapy, family therapy, hospital psychiatry, the management of suicidal patients, child development, and general topics of theoretical interest such as psychoanalytic and psychosocial theory. While these topics continued to be the major emphasis of the program, by the 1990s the conference series also included conferences on more contemporary topics or those for a broad audience beyond the traditional public mental health community.

Topics for CME conferences in the 1990s included: private practice and managed care, suicide prevention, law and psychiatry, AIDS, hypnosis, substance abuse and public policy, psychopharmacology for the nonphysician, children's mental health services, and women's issues. Many of these conferences are now sponsored collaboratively with other institutions such as Wellesley College, McLean Hospital, and the Cambridge Family Institute. Most of the conferences are held under the auspices of Harvard Medical School and speakers include not only department members and other Harvard faculty but also invited guest speakers from throughout the United States. Participants include psychiatrists, psychologists, social workers, nurses, and other therapists, administrators, and academics.

Research Activities

Although, as noted, the Cambridge Hospital is a relatively small (200 bed) community general hospital, it had developed by 1990 a large and established mental health program with a national reputation. Each year some forty interns, psychiatric residents, and child fellows were enrolled in the residency program, as well as over twenty psychology interns and externs who trained there each year. In the 1980s there was a considerable expansion in the program of sponsored research at the department. While this expansion in research was not in itself a manifestation of privatization, it did represent a diversification of funding sources that was significant, and also involved a substantial increase in funding for department activities from philanthropic as well as government sources. Moreover, the nature of the research conducted often can be seen as an extension of the intellectual roots of the departments in the earlier eras of community psychiatry and psychodynamic therapy. It is instructive to review some of these developments.

Much of the research that was developed in the Department of Psychiatry concerned the psychosocial aspects of psychiatry or the delivery of mental health services and the effectiveness of those services. For example, one series of studies supported by the National Institute of Mental Health involved the study of personality disorders and the psychodynamics of individuals with various categories of psychiatric diagnosis. One study examined empirical defense mechanisms and the ways in which patients change through the natural course of their illness or as a result of treatment such as psychotherapy. This type of research was particularly suited to the department's theoretical and clinical orientation. Another set of studies involved the treatment of patients with addictions, including a comparative study of the use of psychotherapy, group therapy, and self-help approaches for the treatment of cocaine addiction. Another study sought to evaluate the effectiveness of preventative measures to reduce the risk of AIDS among intravenous drug users. This research also is grounded in treatment approaches that were well established in the department.

Another set of studies looked at the mental health care system, including hospitals and CMHCs, and attempted to understand the relationship between access to care in public mental hospitals and the changes resulting from deinstitutionalization and privatization. Other research examined the effect of childhood trauma and the later development of severe psychiatric disorders such as schizophrenia and severe personality disorder. Other studies examined the effect of severe psychiatric or substance abuse disorders in mothers on their young children, and followed these children over a period of many years. This research grew out of an interest in child psychiatry and family systems that was prevalent in the department.

These research projects are only a few examples of the many ways in which the academic activities of the department extended into the domain of empirical investigation and psychology and social science studies. These projects often involved several large grants from the federal government or from foundations. The infrastructure for ongoing research was strengthened by the presence of numerous graduate students, research assistants, and consultants and through the publication of scientific papers in professional psychiatric journals. The number of papers published by the faculty now number several hundred per year. The research budget of the organization now accounts for a significant proportion of the total budget, varying from roughly 10 to 20 percent annually.

EPILOGUE

In the 1990s, privatization and entrepreneurial government have become popular philosophies throughout this country and in many other parts of the economically developed world. The application of these approaches in human services, health, and mental health care is transforming the operation of local institutions. Along with the push to privatize has also been a shift toward greater centralization of authority and consolidation of efforts in state government, in universities and medical schools. Purchase of services contracting (described in Chapter 6) is also bringing about restructuring in the scale, scope, and configuration of systems of care. The case of the Cambridge-Somerville Mental Health center illustrates how one local public system has adapted to these trends and pressures and moved in the direction of becoming a blended public-private system. Further developments can be expected as events unfold over the ensuing decade, such as consolidation of state and mental hospitals, increasing use of private general hospitals and introduction of managed care systems both in private and public sectors. These and other future directions are explored in the following chapter of this book.

CHAPTER 8 _____

Future Policy Directions

In this chapter, we will briefly review our earlier discussion of the major components of the mental health care system, before turning to an analysis of the reasons for the failure of some and the success of other mental health systems. In the introduction of this book, we identified four models of care that historically have dominated thinking about the care of the mentally ill in different eras: viewing mental illness as a social abnormality requiring control, viewing mental illness as a long-term disability, viewing it as a condition in need of social service supports, and viewing it as a medical problem. In fact, we believe that these models represent not merely aspects of mental health services, but also subsystems of the health care and social service systems within which mental health services are provided. In many ways, the mental health care system is composed of elements of these larger systems and defined by their intersection or overlapping functions. This is especially true for patients who have severe and chronic conditions, such as schizophrenia, and who are treated primarily in public sector institutions and programs.

Mental health care is strongly influenced by policies set in each of these other external systems. Rather than being able to shape its own policies, mental health systems and organizations are often in the position of responding to those policies set by the other systems, such as health care payment policies, social services regulations, changes in laws governing the criminal justice system, or changes in community zoning regulations. This creates for mental health policymakers, administrators, and practitioners an ever-changing political and economic environment and a sense of ambiguity, confusion, and helplessness. When reforms, policies, or programs "don't work," and are criticized from the perspective of one or another of the large external systems, there may be a perception on the part of the public as well as within the mental health systems of "failure." It is common to read at least annually in major metropolitan newspapers about scandalous events within the public mental health care system. More recently, there have been articles in the national media about poor and unnecessary care in the private mental health services sector as well (Cowley, et al., 1991). This sense of failure can permeate the mental health system and lead to demoralization and paralysis. On the other hand, when the interactions between the sectors are recognized and programs and policies negotiated, there is a possibility of synchronous and constructive efforts. This process may be thought of as striking a balance among competing forces in the mental health system both externally and internally. We believe that understanding better these latent relationships will enable mental health care participants to strengthen policies and practices in order to fulfill their responsibilities to society and ultimately to individual patients. This strengthening would result from greater integration of federal-state policies and more effective implementation at the local community level.

Balance of Models

Bringing balance into the mental health care system involves more than simply prescribing a mix of inputs or products. It requires designing societal and institutional mechanisms for promoting the *integration* of services systems. We have argued that for historical reasons all four basic models of care have an ongoing role in contemporary systems of care; however, it is crucial that attention be paid to maintaining these elements in appropriate balance through explicit policymaking. To incorporate optimally the process of privatization in mental health care systems, for example, involves the integration of institutions (e.g., public and private via contracting); the convergence of philosophies (e.g., introducing notions of market competition to formerly federally-funded CMHCs; and a blurring of categorical focus on patient populations so that all types of needs may be met within a single program (e.g., a general hospital secure admissions unit for evaluation of patients who are young or old, with and without medical comorbidities, insured or uninsured, voluntary or court-mandated, and so forth).

While we propose that there is a need for greater integration of mental health care systems by multiple methods (e.g., case managers, fiscal incentives, family support programs, inter-agency agreements) in order to counter fragmentation, this book has focused on one mechanism, namely, privatization. Privatization, properly implemented, may serve the function of bringing together hitherto disparate parts of the health and mental health system and thereby fostering integration. Alternatively, private companies may fail, which then leads to further problems of discontinuity of treatment, recreating patterns of dysfunction of systems that have plagued mental health systems in the past (Schlesinger, et al., 1986). Controversy and debate continue to surround the issue of privatization for mental health care, with some analysts suggesting it will both raise costs and lower quality (Bass and Locy, 1991).

In implementing privatization, policymakers must contend with what can be referred to as the four Cs: capital, competition, contracting, and capitation. The use of each of these can have a powerful influence in creating institutional incentives to change behavior, to operate efficiently, to be responsive to the needs of clients, and to create new and innovative services. Paradoxically, the arguments espoused by proponents and opponents of privatization tout similar claims. Arguments advanced both for and against privatization are that it leads to: (1) increased or diminished access to care; (2) higher or lower quality of care; (3) less costly or more costly services; (4) more or less community responsiveness and accountability within the system; and (5) greater or lesser administrative efficiency and flexibility. We have seen in our studies presented earlier in this book that the paradoxes stem from a complex reality; for example, access for some patients may be improved at the same time that it may be restricted for others. The problem becomes one not only of whether to privatize— whether government should provide services or should buy services from private contractors—but also how to design and implement privatization, if this approach is selected. This requires a thorough knowledge and understanding of how privatization works and how mental health systems are interrelated and respond to changes.

In the remainder of this chapter, we will elaborate our concept of the roles of the mental health and related systems and the dynamics of their interaction that result in unsuccessful or successful operations. We will discuss each of the aspects of privatization and its potential benefits and risks. We illustrate our analysis with a few examples of recent, apparently successful, reforms in local and state mental health systems—ones that by and large rely on clear principles for successful public policymaking for mental health care. Lastly, we try to look ahead in terms of future directions for services and for research, considering both philosophy and practice, in our attempt to summarize the current state of mental health policy.

Mental Health Systems and Related Systems

A major reason for the lack of integration of mental health systems with other related systems (medical services, long-term care, community social services, and the criminal justice system) is that each of these systems has different traditions, ideologies, and methods for approaching the problems of caring for the mentally ill. We will identify some typical problems that arise when each model is applied to the problems of the mentally ill, discussing both practice models and system policies.

The acute medical care model tends to see illness as episodic, if not random, thus making an insurance approach to paying for care feasible. The physician has a key role to play in making a diagnosis and prescribing a treatment, if not a cure. Viewed in this way, illnesses are time-limited and amenable to intensive treatments, often in a hospital, to be followed by a cure or at least by a period of remission. Modifying social needs is often outside the domain of the immediate caregivers. A significant role is assigned to individual patients to maintain their own well-being and to individual practitioners to provide needed services. Psychiatric care, when viewed as a medical problem, is seen as a discrete product or package of products, and the patient as a consumer who makes informed or "rational" choices. The medical model is designed to address the acute medical needs of patients or, at best, to provide sustained support for subacute medical needs of chronic illnesses that respond to episodic visits to physicians, such as arthritis, hypertension, diabetes, and the like. The medical model is poorly designed to serve the needs of patients with other chronic conditions, such as severe stroke or physical disability, AIDS, or chronic mental illnesses. Patients who require extensive and extended rehabilitation, substantial social supports such as residential care, or who are unable or unwilling to take significant responsibility for their own care are poorly served by most acute care medical systems. Nonetheless, the medical care system does provide insurance coverage (albeit limited), evaluation and management, and acute hospital care for psychiatric patients. As medical systems set standards and policies for the care of psychiatric illnesses, they also influence significantly the "residual" role of public mental health systems, which often also provide intermediate and long-term care for these same individuals.

The long-term care or disability model differs from the acute medical care model in several ways. Needs are defined in terms of providing supportive and rehabilitative services aimed at maintaining or improving social functioning and quality of life. Services are more often provided in a range of community-based settings and may extend to the provision of basic human services, such as housing, transportation, and social activities. A mix of professional inputs is seen as necessary, such as those from psychiatric nurses, social workers, behavioral psychologists, and, more recently, case managers. An example would be a patient who leaves a psychiatric hospital and goes to a halfway house in the community or to a nursing home. The patient may continue to receive psychiatric day-treatment services, make clinic visits for medications, and receive vocational rehabilitation. A case manager may "broker" for the patient the maze of services, medical and social, needed to maintain the individual's functioning outside of a hospital. Federal funding now electively subsidizes case management and rehabilitative services for Medicaid-eligible mentally ill individuals. Case-management services may be performed by an individual who is not trained in any specific mental health profession or discipline, but who nonetheless provides a crucial service for the patient in negotiating treatment through the system. The prototypical disability model in the United States is Social Security Disability Insurance, which provides maintenance supports for individuals who are chronically disabled and who, by definition of eligibility, are unable to work and to be self-supporting. Many of the policies and regulations governing this approach today emanate from the federal government, the most recent being the Americans with Disabilities Act (1991).

The community social services model is epitomized by the community mental health center. In this model, the agency views its responsibility as providing services for a defined geographic community using a population-oriented, not an individual-oriented, approach. Its principal aims are to strengthen communities by providing social services, empower organizations of citizens by vesting them with control of these community services, and focus attention on special at-risk populations. Community services rely heavily on governmental (not insurance-based) financial support. This approach was first institutionalized in the 1960s with the establishment of CMHCs funded for a limited time by the federal government; as the eight-year term of federal support ended, state governments often stepped in to become the primary supporters of these programs, often employing purchase-of-services contracting. Hence, today most policies of community programs are determined by state mental health authorities. In many large cities, multiple centers operate with overlapping jurisdictions and competing local priorities, creating a "patchwork" pattern of services. In addition to state funding for services provided in centers, other sources of funding are often sought, as described in more detail earlier in Chapter 3.

A final model often employed in caring for the mentally ill is that of social control in the form of protective, deterrent, and containing functions, often carried out in institutions. The most widely known of these is the legal mechanism of civil commitment, wherein the individual is detained in a mental hospital against his or her wishes. Specific criteria are applied in determining whether commitment is appropriate, and these criteria usually are contingent on whether or not the individual is judged by professional opinion to be potentially dangerous to himself or others, i.e., suicidal or homicidal. Other forms of intervention are also common, as when individuals who are mentally ill break the law and are imprisoned. In addition, a complex set of standards and regulations has arisen from court cases that have established patients' rights to appropriate treatment. While we usually think of this model of care as applying only to small numbers of individuals, such as those who are determined by the courts to be not guilty by reason of insanity or guilty of crimes of discontrol, such as molestation, in fact the influence of laws and judicial policy toward the mentally ill has had a major impact on the treatment of the mentally ill in society because the main goal of the social control model, since colonial times, has been to secure public safety, rather than to provide therapeutic intervention. The most widely noted examples of the interaction of this control subsystem with the mental health care system have been in a series of "consent decrees" entered into in the last several years between parties suing for adequate care and state governments that have agreed to provide specified packages of services (Okin, 1984). The state must treat patients in the "least restrictive environment" (Geller, et al., 1990). Although improving care for an identified class of claimants, this approach has been criticized for usurping the judgment and discretion of mental health professionals and over time of distorting the budgets and priority-setting of mental health authorities.

Clearly, no single model or perspective is adequate for determining public policy for mentally ill persons; for example, during the institutional era the unsuccessful "monotechnic" solution was asylums or state hospitals. In the 1960s, a romantic fallacy was embodied in thinking that a CMHC could provide mental health care to every person in need, and indeed, to the entire community. Instead, today we must consider how policymaking can proceed with all four models co-existing and interacting with one another, for each model legitimatizes different approaches for its preferred aims. As we consider these different systems—medical, long-term care, social service, and justice—we can see how operational changes in them can influence the mental health care system. We will give some examples from two of these broader systems, although examples could easily be taken from the others as well.

In medical care, there has been a marked increase in corporatization and competition, and growing pressures to contain costs through managed care and utilization review. In the 1980s, state departments of mental health increased contracting for services with private vendors to, for example, manage individual state mental hospitals, to operate community residences, and to provide community aftercare programs. More recently (in 1992), the state of Massachusetts, for example, has contracted with a proprietary health care firm to operate a managed care plan for all Medicaid psychiatric and substance abuse services statewide. These developments, unimagined in the CMHC era of the 1970s, have come about because health care policymakers sanction these approaches to privatization in the 1990s.

At the same time, changes in the long-term care system, such as reforms in Medicaid financing and the introduction of case management systems, also have strongly influenced mental health practices. When federal Medicaid regulations permitted payment for "rehabilitation" services in addition to acute medical care services, state mental health authorities could charge Medicaid for many of the functions of case managers, and both the size and nature of these case management activities grew. Where Medicaid or Medicare pays for services in nursing homes for severely disabled psychiatric patients, patients are moved from mental hospitals to these alternative facilities in a process referred to as "transinstitutionalization." Because Medicaid will pay for day-treatment services, but not hospital care in specialty facilities, patients are now treated in specially designed programs located within the state hospitals so that the facility will be paid for the services provided. Other examples could be cited, but the point is that the mental health care system often reacts to changes in the broader service systems, thereby moving, often suddenly, in one direction or another, but poorly coordinated with the larger medical care systems.

In addition to changes in these broader systems, changes occur simultaneously at two other levels, namely within the mental health care specialty sector and in the government policy environment. Mental health specialty facilities react to broad secular trends and to public perceptions about mental illness and its treatment, and to evolving definitions of what constitutes a mental illness. Today, not only schizophrenia and manic-depressive illnesses are recognized as psychiatric disorders, but so are a host of other conditions now treated in specialty hospitals: substance abuse, eating disorders, post-traumatic stress disorder, conduct disorder of children, chronic pain syndrome, and many more.

The governmental shifts are reflective of broad social and political trends occurring over decades that may shape the structure of mental health programs. We have illustrated some of these governmental shifts in our description, in Chapters 2 and 5, of the CMHC era and the movement toward privatization in the 1980s. We have seen a clear shift over the past decade in view of which level of government should be primarily responsible for social (and mental health care) services; the shift has gone from the federal to the state and, increasingly, to the local unit (e.g., city or county). And we have seen during times of increasing pressures resulting from economic recession and budgetary constraints, an emphasis on individual self-help, on making the family bear the burden of responsibility for care of relatives, and a return to trying to solicit help from volunteers and from philanthropy to provide for the sick and the needy. Mental health systems adapt to the changes in the government's directives. For example, the patient who has Medicaid insurance, and who lives with his or her family, will be expected to receive treatment in short-term, acute care general hospitals (paid for by Medicaid) and to return home to live, even if, in the individual case, a sounder long-term treatment program would be a long stay in a specialty facility (e.g., state mental hospital) and discharge to a community residence with a case manager; such a scenario is illustrated poignantly by the widely reported case of the disjointed "career" as mental patient of Sylvia Frumkin (Moran and Freedman, 1984).

Why Mental Health Systems Fail

There have been many attempts to explain why mental health systems are so often perceived to fail, to be inadequate in meeting the needs of patients, or worse, to be inhumane and harmful. One school of criticism points to the stigma surrounding the mentally ill and to the relative neglect, underfunding, and inattention by states of the needs of the severely mentally ill. This view has most recently been expressed in a series of reports by Torrey, Wolfe, and others under the auspices of the National Alliance for the Mentally Ill and the Public Citizens Health Research Group (Torrey, et al., 1990). They point to the large differences in the amount and types of support for mental health services in different states and report many specific failings of these systems. They blame both societal views and professional norms for the poor condition of many mental health systems. At the same time, they point to examples of success

in many states and help to define the ingredients of such effective programs, suggesting that it is not impossible for local and state efforts to
succeed. Another school of thought about mental health systems focuses
on the internal cycles of reform, and often the dead ends of these cycles.
Many of these studies involve institutional case studies, such as the one
by Morrissey et al. (1980) describing the history and cycles affecting the
Worcester State Hospital. Likewise Talbott (1978) described why the
institutional approach was itself doomed to failure and, noting the long-
standing tensions between institutional and community-oriented ideologies, predicted a trend toward further deinstitutionalization. Among the
broader treatments of this topic of the history of and changes in the mental
health system are those by Grob (1991), which carefully document and
analyze causes of change in policies governing medical care and social
policy. Especially salient in his discussion is the role of professional norms
and treatment practices over time. Often these changes lead to unintended
outcomes, such as the mentally ill who are out of institutions but are now
homeless.

We believe that a major reason why mental health systems fail, and one
of the explanations for the unintended outcomes of reform, lies in the
neglected subject of the nexus of ties of the mental health system with the
other dominant systems described above. It is not simply that mental health
care is a subsystem of health care systems, or of social welfare programs,
but rather that it often functions as a subsidiary or derivative system of
services for all of these others. A recent public relations campaign of the
National Alliance for the Mentally Ill (NAMI), an advocacy group composed of families of the mentally ill, used the motto: "Be a NAMI Wolf"
[not a sheep] to underscore the need for a more assertive stance by the
advocates on behalf of their family members. The mental health care
system, in many local and state jurisdictions, takes on the nature of a
residual system expected somehow to handle the problems not addressed
elsewhere (e.g., what to do about the homeless, the destitute elderly, the
worst addicts, the developmentally disabled, or individuals with AIDS
dementia), creating significant difficulties for ill-prepared mental health
authorities.

The fundamental problem for mental health systems handling these
residual social problems is that policies and practices from the other
broader systems must be implemented; the mental health system cannot
develop a coherent policy of its own. The basic mission of the mental
health authority is diffused as it incorporates elements of the missions of
other systems. [We hasten to add that we are not advocating that policies
should be developed solely within mental health agencies, rather that

better processes be developed for working with the external systems, for example, through interagency agreements.]

Another problem is that the target or priority population to be served is so heterogeneous as to be ill-defined and potentially expandable. This dispersion of responsibilities makes difficult the setting of policies and the selection of professional expertise needed to treat the patients. Ultimately, it can lead to dilution of resources in a variety of directions in an attempt to meet all the needs of a varied group of people. So, one will find mental health authorities in various jurisdictions with primary responsibility not only for the treatment of the severely mentally ill but also operating a host of institutions and programs: homeless shelters, AIDS hospices, drug treatment programs, nursing homes [skilled nursing facilities], prison units, foster care for children, schools for adolescents, medical units for psychiatric patients, housing projects, and so on.

It is questionable whether the state mental health authority is the best equipped agency to operate these alternative programs. In some states, the recognition that these programs are not really within the technical expertise of the mental health agency leads the agency to contract with outside providers and to pay for the identified services with funds from the mental health agency budget. Although this may be a rational management approach to the problem of how best to provide the service in question, it begs the more basic policy issue of whether it is primarily the responsibility (within the context of state or local government) of the mental health system to provide these services.

Although it may be true that the public mental health system, for a variety of social historical reasons (including stigmatization), has generally less legitimacy and authority (and related funding constraints) than some other branches of government, there remain a set of problems specifically associated with the transmission of policies from the larger systems to the mental health system that influence mental health care, and which should be addressed. Mental health systems, because of their size, role, authority, and influence, may be particularly vulnerable to these external pressures. One illustration would be the size and scope of the federal mental health agency (the National Institute of Mental Health, NIMH) within the federal government. Although the expenditures by the federal government through various venues for mental health care amount to several billion dollars, the budget of the NIMH is less than $1 billion annually, with most of that devoted to basic research. At the state level, it is often noted that mental health commissioners are difficult to recruit, have short (average) tenure in their positions (less than two years), and reportedly occupy politically and managerially stressful positions, often

becoming an object of public criticism, legislative scrutiny, and professional hostility. Rather than focus on purported managerial deficiencies,
however, let us consider some of the systems dynamics alluded to earlier
in this chapter that form the management matrix for mental health agencies.

Balance of Systems

Changes in the external systems exert a pull on mental health policies
in different directions and at different rates, resulting in dislocations,
distortions and imbalances in the core mental health sector. Because of a
customary natural degree of bureaucratic and institutional inertia, efforts
to exert pressure for change in any given direction often result in strain,
stress and tensions. For example, the overburdened criminal justice system
may exert pressure on the mental health care system to treat greater
numbers of violent so-called "criminally insane," but the mental health
system may resist the shifts in responsibility and in fact may not have
suitable facilities and staff sufficient to adapt quickly to such a mandate.

In another example, a mayor or governor may decide to respond to
public concern about homeless mentally ill by directing the social services
agency to use mental health authority facilities to open large-scale residential programs for these individuals; however, such an initiative may
run afoul of civil rights concerns, of public health department regulations
governing the use of hospitals, or of mental health plans for reducing
residential populations and shifting staffing resources to the community
(in part to reach out to homeless persons). At a minimum there will be the
inevitable disputes about allocation of funds for the new and more expensive programs; not because housing *per se* is so expensive, but because
the need for staffing, heating, feeding, providing transportation, security,
health care, and ancillary services readily becomes evident. In the absence
of a coherent mental health policy and mandate, the mental health system
quickly may be seen as "out of synch" with the other systems, even when
its leaders may agree with the proposed external changes and wish to be
cooperative and responsive.

At other times, the pulls from external systems may be contradictory,
that is, changes in one of the external systems may pull mental health
services policy in one direction, while change in another system pulls it
in another. Such paradoxes are inherent in public policy toward health and
welfare services and are both predictable and unavoidable. At a time when
pressure is being exerted to reduce acute care hospital capacity, there is a
burgeoning of new hospitals and units for psychiatric services. To illustrate

the dilemma with a current example, while there continues to be an emphasis on client choice within acute medical care, there is an increased emphasis on case management and limiting choice in long-term care. Mental health policy may either be paralyzed and caught between equal countervailing pressures, or it may be pulled in opposite directions simultaneously. Should the homeless mentally ill be viewed as a problem for the mental health agencies or the social services and housing agencies? Often the mental health system, aware of the importance of its ties to related external systems, will attempt to adapt to both sets of requirements, leading to ambiguity or fragmentation for the system and confusion and inconsistencies for providers, clients, and families.

It is much easier to identify the sources of potential friction and inappropriate transmission of policy directives than it is to identify generalizable strategies for coping with these problems. One reason is that states differ so markedly in the administrative structures of their mental health authorities. Another is that the external systems in these states also historically have structures and missions that vary from one locale to another. Even within large states, governing structures and relationships for mental health systems differ. Nonetheless the general problem we wish to emphasize is the inappropriate, or at least uncoordinated, transmission of the larger systems' policies to mental health care programs. This results in a sense among the mental health care community of being the followers, rather than leading the way in setting policy for groups of vulnerable people with special needs.

For administrators struggling to coordinate policy in such a complex environment, there are probably several strategies that may be useful. Trying to control the rate of transmission of policies or to reduce the lag time in responding to appropriate policies by speeding up the internal response time of the agency may be helpful. The mental health authority management team would function as a filter to screen, digest, and tailor policies affecting mental health programs before transmitting them to others in the system. At times it may be necessary to alter the relationships with external systems and to realign mental health services of different sorts with specific external systems. For example, when the problems of relating the needs of the mentally ill and the mentally retarded within a single agency in Massachusetts appeared to become a major obstacle to progress for both constituencies, the Department of Mental Health was divided into separate departments, one for mental health and one for mental retardation. On the other hand, in some other states, such an approach might not make sense because of the size of the departments and relative scarcity of fiscal, managerial, technical, human, and institutional resources available for serving the different groups.

The major approaches to addressing the problems we have identified must involve reform of macrosystems that address the need for better coordination and integration of care. We have focused on privatization as one such systemic approach that is being widely used by many states today. Other approaches, some also involving aspects of privatization, focusing on management reform or on changing our perspectives on long-term goals for the severely and persistently mentally ill, should be noted. Many of these approaches are described elsewhere in much more detail and are widely available to interested readers (Shore and Cohen, 1990). We make no claim that privatization should be the primary direction of policy reform, but rather that it is one direction that is being widely used and one that meets the criteria of cutting across the systems boundaries and potentially integrating heretofore separate systems of care. It is, as our extensive studies of the phenomenon demonstrate, no panacea; however, as was the case with deinstitutionalization, it appears to be a megatrend that will have a major influence on the financing and delivery of mental health services for a long time to come. It therefore deserves to be the subject of rigorous analysis and study as to its impact, both positive and unintended.

Need for Integration of Mental Health Systems

When we view mental health systems from the perspective of how other social systems function, certain critical issues emerge as being of primary importance. One of these is *integration*. A social system perspective has been applied extensively to the study of psychiatric hospitals, community mental health centers and community organizations. Marcus and Edelson (1967) identify four major functions of mental health systems: (1) direct treatment; (2) distribution of resources; (3) education; and (4) integration. They suggest that of these, integration is the "most neglected and most important" one but that it may be a superordinate function, coordinating public-private, federal-state, institution-community dimensions of a mental health system. It may be viewed as organizing the organizations, with special emphasis on ensuring continuity of care for individuals. In considering how privatization, or any other major trend in mental health policy, contributes to performance of the systems of care, we should pay particular attention to how it influences the integration of treatment programs. Specifically, we should be concerned about how it affects the following aspects of performance: (1) access to care; (2) treatment capacity and quality; (3) community integration and accountability; and (4) systems economics and costs.

The four Cs of privatization mentioned earlier in this chapter—capital, competition, contracting, and capitation—represent recent approaches to reform of mental health systems by introducing financial mechanisms that foster integration through privatization. Capital refers to the use of private sector incentives and finances that bring additional funds into the construction and operation of new psychiatric hospitals. One example of the use of capital is the construction of several new psychiatric teaching hospitals in joint ventures with universities and medical schools. Construction of facilities has also occurred in rural areas where none existed previously.

Competition in a traditional market structure is argued to be desirable for bringing about efficiencies of management and lower costs, and innovation and quality assurance. As we have seen, the results of competition in psychiatric care have been mixed. In some geographic areas where there had been no psychiatric hospitals, several were established simultaneously, leading to an oversupply of beds, when state certificate-of-need laws designed to discourage excess hospital growth expired. In some areas, this expansion has led to over-capacity that pushed some hospitals into treating more poor patients than they would otherwise have accepted, such as those with Medicaid or those referred by CMHCs. It has also resulted in much greater capacity for treating adolescents but, according to critics, it has also led to some unnecessary treatment of those with insurance.

Contracting for services by state governments seeks to take advantage of the flexibility of the private sector to respond to the changing needs of local areas. By specifying what services are to be provided, the funding agency can more efficiently utilize its resources, it is argued. Costs for contracted services in private facilities are often lower than in state funded facilities, especially at first, because salaries offered by private vendors may be lower and there may be lower overhead costs than in large, bureaucratic public organizations. In a competitive environment, bidders are forced to minimize the price they charge and ideally, to maximize the quality of services offered. (We have elsewhere noted a number of problems that may arise when the market is not functioning ideally, or competition is minimal.) Other problems arise as vendors grow into mega-vendors beset by many of the same problems affecting large public organizations: increasing overhead costs, unionized employees, financial and performance accountability problems.

Capitation is only beginning to be a factor in mental health care as managed care programs for patients formerly treated in the public sector are introduced by insurance providers. A number of capitation experiments are underway in various local systems (e.g., cities, catchment areas, counties, or in a limited way in a few states). This latter aspect of privatization brings to the fore one of the basic tenets of another school of thought concerning needed reforms in public mental health systems, namely, the "central authority" approach. The central authority is best described and illustrated by the Robert Wood Johnson Foundation's national nine-city demonstration program for the care of the chronically mentally ill (Shore and Cohen, 1990).

We believe all of these efforts have in common, either explicitly or implicitly, the goal of increasing the integration of the mental health care system with other health and human services systems. Explicitly included in many privatization proposals is the movement of care from state mental hospitals to community general hospitals (Fisher, et al., 1992), a sort of "mainstreaming" of mental health care. A second major direction is the integration of mental health services with social services through the use of Medicare (disability) benefits and specially-designated housing services. This integration is fostered by using case managers who interface between the mental health and social service systems on behalf of mentally ill patients. Another type of integration is occurring through the use of contracts between state governments and community mental health centers that pay for services not for the entire community but rather for specific patients who meet predetermined criteria of major mental illness. In some states, such as Massachusetts, Wisconsin, and Ohio, all of these developments of privatization linking mental health care to medical, social, and community services are taking place simultaneously, thereby drawing the sectors into closer collaboration. In some instances, this tightening of relationships is the result of deliberate reform-oriented planning (e.g., Ohio) while in others it appears to be driven by declining budgets and the need to increase efficiency (e.g., Massachusetts). Where financial incentives have been directly related to critical key performance measures, such as reducing the rates of admission to hospitals by use of community alternatives, there has been notable success both in bringing about balancing of the system and in increasing public satisfaction with system performance (Taube, et al., 1990).

CONCLUSION

Recently, the National Institute of Mental Health (NIMH, 1991; 1992) has identified a number of important directions and innovations believed by their staff and expert consultants to hold the most promise for improving the care for people with severe mental disorders. In the area of clinical services, they identified the following areas as being of critical importance: (1) improved diagnostic assessment and measurement of disability and quality of life; (2) enhanced integration, continuity and quality of care; (3) introduction of rehabilitation programs involving social skills, vocational training, and consumer and family orientations; and (4) focus on long-term outcomes in multiple domains, including social services as well as medical. In the area of service systems organization and financing of care, they stressed the need for improving services systems at the local level, especially by matching local services to needs. New concepts and methods in organizational research were suggested to improve integration of care.

We would agree with these approaches and have further emphasized the need to coordinate financing from public and private sources to cover acute and chronic service needs for patients and former patients. Against this backdrop, privatization takes on enormous importance, both for its potential to integrate public and private services and because it may make better use of available financing through a variety of creative arrangements for supporting mental health services. There remains, however, a crucial role for public authorities to fund, monitor, and regulate the provision of services to the poorest, most vulnerable, and disenfranchised among the seriously and persistently mentally ill. As we move into a new era of national health care reform based on approaches such as "managed competition," the lessons of privatization of mental health care can help to improve future mental health policies.

Appendix:
Study Instrument—Questionnaire

THE NATIONAL MENTAL HEALTH FACILITIES STUDY

SECTION A. HOSPITAL BACKGROUND DATA

1. Name of person completing this questionnaire _____

2. Title _____

3. Hospital Name_____

4. Your hospital's most recently completed fiscal year began on:

   month_____ day_____ year_____ and ended on month_____ day_____ year_____

5. Please check *one* box to indicate the type of organization that is responsible for the operation of this hospital.

   FOR PROFIT   NONPROFIT   STATE/LOCAL GOVERNMENT

   ☐ 1 Individual   ☐ 4 Religious organization   ☐ 6 State government

   ☐ 2 Partnership   ☐ 5 Other nonprofit   ☐ 7 County government

   ☐ 3 Corporation   ☐ 8 City government

                                                                 ☐ 10 District or regional authority

6. How long has your facility been operating under the current ownership?

                                                                 _____ years

7. Is your hospital owned or managed by another organization?

                                                                 ☐ 1 Owned

                                                                 ☐ 2 Managed

                                                                 ☐ 3 Neither

8. If the hospital is owned or managed by another organization, please print the name of the organization:

   _____

GENERAL HOSPITALS ONLY: PLEASE ANSWER QUESTIONS #9 THROUGH #11.
ALL OTHERS SKIP TO QUESTION #12.

9. Is the psychiatric unit owned or managed by an organization other than the owner of the hospital?

                                                                 ☐ 1 Owned

                                                                 ☐ 2 Managed

                                                                 ☐ 3 Neither

10. If the unit is owned or managed by another organization, please print the name of the organization:

    _____

11. Is this organization operated as a for-profit or nonprofit corporation?

                                                                 ☐ 1 For-profit

                                                                 ☐ 2 Nonprofit

---

12. What is the *total* number of beds set up and staffed at your facility?

_____ beds

13. How many beds do you have set up and staffed for psychiatric care?
(PLEASE DO NOT INCLUDE SCATTER BEDS.)

_____ beds

14. How many of these beds are in the following specialized units?

Number of Beds

a. Separate children and adolescent units . . . . _____

b. Separate geriatrics unit . . . . _____

c. Separate alcoholism and/or substance abuse unit . . . . . . _____

d. Separate eating disorders unit . . . . _____

15. Do you have an accredited psychiatric residency program?

☐ 1 Yes

☐ 2 No

16. In the last month, what was the average daily census for psychiatric inpatients at your facility?

_____ (number)

SECTION B.   SOURCES OF PATIENTS

1. Service Area: Which *best* describes the area from which your hospital regularly serves patients?
(PLEASE CHECK ONLY ONE RESPONSE.)

a. City or county in which your facility is located . . . . ☐

b. County and contiguous counties . . . . ☐

c. State in which your facility is located . . . . ☐

d. State and contiguous states . . . . ☐

e. Nation . . . . ☐

2. What percent of your *inpatients* come to your facility from each of the following referral sources?

(PLEASE CHECK ONE FOR EACH SOURCE.)

Sources	Percent		
	0-5%	6-20%	21+%
a. Private practitioner	☐	☐	☐
b. Private psychiatric hospital	☐	☐	☐
c. Public psychiatric hospital	☐	☐	☐
d. General hospital inpatient units	☐	☐	☐
e. General hospital emergency rooms	☐	☐	☐
f. Community Mental Health Centers	☐	☐	☐
g. Employee Assistance Plans	☐	☐	☐
h. Health Maintenance Organizations	☐	☐	☐
i. Social service agencies and courts	☐	☐	☐
j. Self-referred	☐	☐	☐

3. Which of the following characterizes the relationship between your hospital and the referral sources? Is there a formal agreement, an informal agreement, or no agreement to refer patients?

(PLEASE CHECK ALL THAT APPLY.)

Sources	Formal written agreement(s)	Informal or verbal agreement(s)	No agreement
a. Private practitioner	1 ☐	2 ☐	0 ☐
b. Private psychiatric hospital	1 ☐	2 ☐	0 ☐
c. Public psychiatric hospital...............	1 ☐	2 ☐	0 ☐
d. General hospital inpatient units..........	1 ☐	2 ☐	0 ☐
e. General hospital emergency rooms	1 ☐	2 ☐	0 ☐
f. Community Mental Health Centers	1 ☐	2 ☐	0 ☐
g. Employee Assistance Plans	1 ☐	2 ☐	0 ☐
h. Health Maintenance Organizations.......	1 ☐	2 ☐	0 ☐
i. Social service agencies and courts	1 ☐	2 ☐	0 ☐
j. Self-referred	1 ☐	2 ☐	0 ☐

SECTION C. CONTRACTS AND AFFILIATIONS

1. Does your hospital or parent corporation *own* any of the following?
(PLEASE CIRCLE CORRECT RESPONSE FOR EACH.)

	YES	NO
a. HMOs and PPOs	1	2
b. Residential care facilities	1	2
c. Community Mental Health Centers	1	2
d. Outpatient offices	1	2
e. Home health care agencies	1	2
f. Nursing homes	1	2

2. Does your hospital have a *contract* or *joint venture* with any of the following?
(PLEASE CIRCLE AS MANY AS APPLY.)

	Contract	Joint Venture	Neither
a. Physician groups	1	2	0
b. HMOs and PPOs	1	2	0
c. Private psychiatric facilities	1	2	0
d. Residential care facilities	1	2	0
e. Clinics/Community Mental Health Centers	1	2	0
f. Home health care agencies	1	2	0
g. Emergency rooms of general hospitals	1	2	0
h. Nursing homes	1	2	0

3.1 In your last fiscal year, has your hospital provided mental health care services under contract to state, county or city government agencies?

□ 1 Yes

□ 2 No

3.2 If you have provided any of the following services under contract, please circle the method(s) of payment used for each.

(PLEASE CIRCLE AS MANY AS APPLY.)

	METHOD(S) OF PAYMENT			
	Fee for service	Fixed Sum Budget	Fee per patient (e.g. capitation)	No Contract
a. Inpatient services	1	2	3	0
b. Day treatment services or partial hospitalization	1	2	3	0
c. Consultation and education	1	2	3	0
d. Emergency psychiatric services	1	2	3	0
e. Case management services	1	2	3	0

SECTION D: SELECTED MENTAL HEALTH SERVICES

1. Below are *selected* psychiatric services sometimes offered by hospitals. In the last year, did your facility offer or contract for any of the following services?

(PLEASE CIRCLE CORRECT RESPONSE.)

	YES	NO
a. Geriatric psychiatry	1	2
b. Outpatient psychiatric clinics or therapist offices	1	2
c. 24 hour emergency psychiatric services	1	2
d. Residential psychiatric treatment facilities or halfway houses	1	2
e. Case management for chronically mentally ill	1	2
f. Telephone hotline or suicide prevention	1	2

2. How many *other* health care facilities located within 15 miles of your hospital offered this service in the last year?

(PLEASE CHECK THE CORRECT RESPONSE FOR EACH.)

a. Geriatric psychiatry	0 □	1 □	2-5 □	5+ □
b. Outpatient psychiatric clinics or therapist offices	0 □	1 □	2-5 □	5+ □
c. 24 hour emergency psychiatric services	0 □	1 □	2-5 □	5+ □
d. Residential psychiatric treatment facilities or halfway houses	0 □	1 □	2-5 □	5+ □
e. Case management for chronically mentally ill	0 □	1 □	2-5 □	5+ □
f. Telephone hotline or suicide prevention	0 □	1 □	2-5 □	5+ □

SECTION E. SERVICE ENVIRONMENT

IN THIS SECTION PLEASE CIRCLE THE NUMBER THAT MOST CLOSELY APPLIES.

1. To what extent must your hospital compete with other facilities to attract patients for *inpatient* psychiatric care?

Not at All		Some Extent		Great Extent
1	2	3	4	5

2. To what extent must your hospital compete with other facilities to attract *outpatients* for care at your hospital?

Do Not Treat Outpatients ☐	Not at All		Some Extent		Great Extent
	1	2	3	4	5

3. In the past year, has your hospital done any of the following:

	Not at All		Some Extent		A great Extent
a. Direct marketing to potential patients	1	2	3	4	5
b. Reduced non-physician clinical staff	1	2	3	4	5
c. Reduced administrative staff	1	2	3	4	5
d. Encouraged the use of short-term treatment	1	2	3	4	5
f. Added services to encourage admissions	1	2	3	4	5
g. Reduced charges	1	2	3	4	5
h. Eliminated marginally profitable services	1	2	3	4	5

4. How much influence do each of the following persons or groups have in formulating specific areas of management or policy affecting psychiatric patients in your hospital?

	A. Adding psychiatric services			B. Setting annual budget			C. Developing clinical policies		
	Very Little	Some	Very Much	Very Little	Some	Very Much	Very Little	Some	Very Much
a. Hospital administrator	1	2	3	1	2	3	1	2	3
b. Chief of service/Medical staff	1	2	3	1	2	3	1	2	3
c. Central corporate office	1	2	3	1	2	3	1	2	3
d. Hospital Board of Directors	1	2	3	1	2	3	1	2	3
e. Third party payors (including Medicare/Medicaid)	1	2	3	1	2	3	1	2	3
f. CMHCs or other local human service agencies	1	2	3	1	2	3	1	2	3
g. State agencies	1	2	3	1	2	3	1	2	3
h. Citizen advocacy group	1	2	3	1	2	3	1	2	3

SECTION F. PATIENT CHARACTERISTICS

1. Please enter the *percent of inpatients* treated in your hospital in the last year for each of the following primary diagnoses.

Principal DSM-III Diagnosis	Percent
a. Affective disorders	_____%
b. Anxiety/somatic disorders	_____%
c. Schizophrenia and other psychotic disorders	_____%
d. Personality disorder	_____%
e. Alcoholism	_____%
f. Other substance abuse	_____%
g. Organic mental disorder (includes Alzheimer's Disease)	_____%
h. Disorders of childhood and adolescence	_____%
i. No mental disorder	_____%
	100%

2. In the past fiscal year, what percent of total psychiatric patient care revenues at your hospital came from the following sources?

Payor	Patient Care Revenues
a. Blue Cross/Blue Shield	_____%
b. Commercial Insurance	_____%
c. Medicare	_____%
d. Medicaid	_____%
e. Self-pay	_____%
f. HMOs/PPOs	_____%
g. Contracts with county and state	_____%
	100%

3. In your last fiscal year, what percent of your psychiatric patient charges were not collected?

(PLEASE DO NOT INCLUDE DISCOUNTS OR CONTRACTUAL ALLOWANCES.)

Inpatient: _____%

Outpatient: _____%

4. In your last fiscal year, for what percent of psychiatric patients did you offer care at reduced charge?

(PLEASE INCLUDE SLIDING FEES. DO NOT INCLUDE HMO/PPO DISCOUNTS.)

Inpatient: _____%

Outpatient: _____%

5. In your last fiscal year, did your institution set a minimum percentage of its budget to be spent on uncompensated psychiatric care?

☐ 1 Yes

☐ 2 No

6. When funds for uncompensated care are exhausted, which of the following *best* describes the policies that are adopted to limit further costs for uninsured patients?

(PLEASE CHECK ONLY ONE RESPONSE.)

a. No change in admitting practices. ☐

b. Patients without insurance are admitted on a case by case basis, with review by hospital administration. ☐

c. Patients are admitted only under emergency conditions, their conditions are stabilized, and they are discharged. ☐

d. Staff and attending physicians are advised about budgetary conditions and requested not to admit uninsured patients. ☐

e. A moratorium is established on uncompensated care for the rest of the year. ☐

SECTION G.   STAFF AND STAFFING POLICIES

1. Staff *employed* by your hospital in the past year:

Category of Staff	Number of Full-Time Equivalent Employees
a. Psychiatrists	_____ (number)
b. Psychologists (PhD)	_____ (number)
c. Social Workers (MSW)	_____ (number)
d. Registered Nurses (include MSN)	_____ (number)
e. Licensed Practical Nurses	_____ (number)
f. Other mental health workers (BA)	_____ (number)
g. Other mental health workers (non-BA)	_____ (number)
h. Trainees (residents and interns)	_____ (number)

2.1 Private practitioners *(not hospital employees)* treating inpatients at your hospital:

	Number Who Treated Patients in Last Month
a. Psychiatrists	_____ (number)
b. Psychologists	_____ (number)

2.2 Please estimate the *average number of hours* of inpatient care provided in a typical week by each private practitioner who admits patients to your hospital:

_____ hours

3. Do any psychiatrists receive incentive payments based on the overall economic performance of your hospital or psychiatric unit?

(PLEASE CHECK ALL THAT APPLY.)

☐ 1 Yes, staff psychiatrists

☐ 2 Yes, private practitioners

☐ 3 None

4. Please estimate the turnover rate in the past year in your facility for:
(TURNOVER RATE = STAFF TERMINATIONS DIVIDED BY TOTAL STAFF OF THAT TYPE.)

registered nurses _____% TURNOVER

mental health workers (non BA) _____% TURNOVER

SECTION H.   MONITORING TREATMENT POLICIES

1. How often does the *primary* responsibility for assuring that aftercare services are received by patients rest with:

	Never	Sometimes	Often
a. Patient............................	1	2	3
b. Private practitioner	1	2	3
c. State or community agency other than this hospital.............	1	2	3
d. This hospital's staff..................	1	2	3

2. After formal discharge plans are prepared for a patient and before the patient leaves the hospital, is the plan reviewed by a treatment team?

☐ 1 Yes

☐ 2 No

3. Which of the following *most closely* describes the procedure your facility uses for monitoring patients' aftercare?

(PLEASE CHECK ONLY ONE.)

a. Patient is given appointment at community agency ....☐

b. Telephone contact person is available at your hospital to help patient with referral ....☐

c. Following discharge, a letter is sent to the patient reminding him/her of outpatient appointment ....☐

d. One or more phone calls to outpatient provider to assure patient has kept first outpatient appointment ....☐

e. A designated hospital staff member visits outpatient clinics regularly to follow up discharged patients......☐

f. One or more visits to patient's residence if unable to reach patient by phone..........................☐

4. Is there a particular staff member or department at your facility whose primary responsibility is assuring that a patient's aftercare is provided?

☐ 1 Yes

☐ 2 No

5. On average, for how long a time does your facility monitor patient status after discharge?

(PLEASE CHECK ONLY ONE.)

a. up to 1 week ....☐

b. up to 1 month............☐

c. up to 6 months ....☐

d. up to 1 year..............☐

6. In order to monitor care in your facility, do you use any of the following methods?

	YES	NO
a. Patient satisfaction questionnaire	1	2
b. Utilization review committee	1	2
c. Monitoring use of medications	1	2
d. Physical examination by primary care physician	1	2
e. Patient grievance procedure	1	2
f. Review of length of stay assignment	1	2
g. Review short-term readmission rates to your facility	1	2
h. Patient rights advocate	1	2
i. Review of accidents and violent incidents	1	2
j. Suicide review conferences	1	2
k. Monitoring use of restraint and/or seclusion	1	2
l. Internal review of appropriateness of admission	1	2

7.1 To what extent do you believe JCAH standards contribute to quality of care in psychiatric facilities?

Not at all		Some extent		Great extent
1	2	3	4	5

7.2 Is your institution accredited by JCAH?

☐ 1 Yes

☐ 2 No

SECTION I. ATTITUDES ABOUT THE MENTAL HEALTH CARE SYSTEM

Please think about how strongly you agree or disagree with each of the following statements.
(RATE EACH STATEMENT BY CIRCLING THE APPROPRIATE NUMBER ON THE FIVE POINT SCALE.)

1. The role of the administrator is to ensure that support services are provided to the clinical staff without influencing clinical practice.

Strongly Agree	Agree	Undecided	Disagree	Strongly Disagree
1	2	3	4	5

2. The board of directors of a psychiatric hospital should ensure that hospital services meet the mental health needs of the local community.

Strongly Agree	Agree	Undecided	Disagree	Strongly Disagree
1	2	3	4	5

3. Identifying all unmet mental health needs in the community should be the responsibility of government agencies rather than psychiatric hospitals.

Strongly Agree	Agree	Undecided	Disagree	Strongly Disagree
1	2	3	4	5

4. Patients with insurance should indirectly pay for the care of uninsured patients.

Strongly Agree	Agree	Undecided	Disagree	Strongly Disagree
1	2	3	4	5

5. Paying economic incentives (such as bonuses) to clinical staff may compromise appropriate standards of care.

Strongly Agree	Agree	Undecided	Disagree	Strongly Disagree
1	2	3	4	5

6. A private facility cannot be expected to offer a service if the revenues for that service do not exceed costs.

Strongly Agree	Agree	Undecided	Disagree	Strongly Disagree
1	2	3	4	5

7. Paying economic incentives (such as bonuses) to clinical staff is necessary to encourage clinicians to efficiently deliver psychiatric services.

Strongly Agree	Agree	Undecided	Disagree	Strongly Disagree
1	2	3	4	5

8. Please rank in order of importance from 1 (most important) to 5 (least important) the following factors as indicators of quality care in inpatient psychiatric facilities:

	Rank
a. Well-trained professional staff	_____
b. Adequate numbers of professional and non-professional staff	_____
c. Modern well-equipped facilities	_____
d. A dedicated and caring attitude on the part of patient-care staff	_____
e. A high level of patient satisfaction	_____

Please use this space or an additional sheet to elaborate on any of the information supplied on this form. If you have any printed material that you believe will be helpful, such as your annual report, please enclose it with the questionnaire, in the accompanying prepaid envelope.

_____

_____

_____

_____

_____

Thank you very much for your cooperation.

References

Adams EK, Ellwood MH, Pine PL. Utilization and expenditures under Medicaid for Supplemental Security Income disabled. *Health Care Financing Review* II(1):1–24, 1989.

American Psychiatric Association (APA). *Economic Fact Book for Psychiatry*. Washington, DC: American Psychiatric Press, 1989.

Anthony WA, Buell GJ, Sharratt S, Althoff ME. Efficacy of psychiatric rehabilitation. *Psychological Bulletin* 78:447–56, 1972.

Babigian HM, Marshall PE. Rochester: A comprehensive capitation experiment. In, *Paying for Services: Promises and Pitfalls of Capitation*. Mechanic D and Aiken LH (Eds). San Francisco: Jossey-Bass, 1989, pp. 43–54.

Barton WE. *The History and Influence of the American Psychiatric Association*. Washington, DC: American Psychiatric Press, 1986.

Bass A, Locy T. New policies hit the mentally ill. *Boston Globe* Dec 15, 1991, p. 1.

Beers CW. *A Mind That Found Itself*. Pittsburgh, PA: University of Pittsburgh Press, 1981; reprint of 1907 original.

Berman N, Hoppe EW. Halfway house residents: where do they go? *J Community Psychology* 4:259–60, 1976.

Bloche MG, Cournos F. Mental health policy for the 1990s: tinkering in the interstices. *J Health Politics Policy Law* 2: 387–411, 1990.

Bockoven JS. *Moral Treatment in Community Mental Health*. New York: Springer, 1972.

Bok D. *Beyond the Ivory Tower: Social Responsibilities of the Modern University*. Cambridge, MA: Harvard University Press, 1982.

Borenstein DB. Managed care: A means of rationing psychiatric treatment. *Hosp Community Psychiatry* 41:1095–98, 1990.

Brady J, Sharfstein S, Muszynski I. Trends in private insurance coverage for mental illness. *Am J Psychiatry* 143:1276–79, 1986.

Brown P (Ed). *Mental Health Care and Social Policy*. Boston: Rutledge & Kegan Paul, 1985.

Carling PJ. Major mental illness, housing and supports: the promise of community integration. *Am Psychologist* 45:969–75, 1990.

Carter R. *The Accountable Agency*. Beverly Hills, CA: Sage Publications, 1983.

Castel R, Castel F, Lovell A. *The Psychiatric Society*. New York: Columbia University Press, 1982.

Chu FD, Trotter S. *The Madness Establishment: Ralph Nader's Study Group Report on the NIMH*. New York: Grossman, 1974.

City of Cambridge. *First Annual Report*. 1917.

Clark RE, Dorwart RA. Competition and CMHAs. *J Health Politics Policy Law*. 17: 517–40, 1992.

Cotton PG, Bene-Kociemba A, Cole R. The effect of deinstitutionalization on a general hospital's inpatient psychiatric service. *Hosp Community Psychiatry* 30:609–12, 1979.

Cowley G, et al. Money madness. *Newsweek* Nov 4, 1991, pp. 50–52.

Cromwell J, Harrow B, McGuire TG, Ellis RP. Medicare payment to psychiatric facilities. *Health Aff (Millwood)* 10(2):124–34, 1991.

Dain N. *Concepts of Insanity in the U.S., 1789–1865*. New Brunswick, NJ: Rutgers University Press, 1964.

Davidson H, Schlesinger M, Dorwart RA, Schnell E. State purchase of mental health care: models and motivations for maintaining accountability. *Intl J Law Psychiatry* 14:387–403, 1991.

DeHoog RH. *Contracting Out for Human Services: Economic, Political, and Organizational Perspectives*. Albany, NY: State University of New York Press, 1984.

Deutsch A. *The Mentally Ill in America, 2nd Ed*. New York: Columbia University Press, 1949.

Deutsch A. *The Shame of the States*. New York: Harcourt Brace, 1948.

Dix DL. *Memorial*. Boston: Munroe and Francis, 1843.

Dobson A, Scharff-Corder L. Six months of Medicaid data. *Health Care Financing Review* 4:115–21, 1983.

Donahue JD. *The Privatization Decision: Public Ends, Private Means*. New York: Basic Books, 1989.

Dorwart RA. Innovation or irregulars: homeopathy and psychiatry, Westborough State Hospital, 1886–1986. *Psychiatric News* April 7, 1989, p. 17.

Dorwart RA. Managed mental health care: myths and realities in the 1990's. *Hosp Community Psychiatry* 41:1087–91, 1990.

Dorwart RA. A ten-year follow-up study of the effects of deinstitutionalization. *Hosp Community Psychiatry* 39:287–91, 1988.

Dorwart RA, Chartock LR. Psychiatry and the resource-based relative value scale. *Am J Psychiatry* 145:1237–42, 1988.

Dorwart RA, Chartock LR, Dial T, et al. A national study of psychiatrists' professional activities. *Am J Psychiatry* 149: 1499–1505, 1992a.

Dorwart RA, Epstein SS. Economics and mental health care: the HMO as a crucible for cost-effective care. In, *Managed Mental Health Care.* Fitzpatrick R, Feldman J (Eds). Washington, DC: APPI, 1992.

Dorwart RA, Epstein SS. Issues in psychiatric hospital care. *Current Opinion Psychiatry* 4:789–93, 1991.

Dorwart RA, Epstein SS, Chartock L. Financing of services. In, *Textbook of Administrative Psychiatry.* Talbott JT, Hales RE, Keill SL (Eds). Washington, DC: American Psychiatric Press, Inc., 1992b.

Dorwart RA, Schlesinger M. Privatization of psychiatric services. *Am J Psychiatry* 145:543–53, 1988.

Dorwart RA, Schlesinger M, Davidson H, Epstein SS, Hoover C. A national study of psychiatric hospital care. *Am J Psychiatry* 148:204–10, 1991.

Eisenberg L. The case against for-profit hospitals. *Hosp Community Psychiatry* 35:1009–13, 1984.

Ermann D, Gabel J. Multihospital systems: issues and empirical findings. *Health Aff (Millwood)* 3(1):50–64, 1984.

Estes CL, Wood JB. A preliminary assessment of the impact of block grants on community mental health centers. *Hosp Community Psychiatry* 35:1125–29, 1984.

Feis CL, Mowbray CT, Chamberlain PJ. Serving the chronic mentally ill in state and community hospitals. *Community Mental Health J* 26:221–32, 1990.

Felix RH. A model of comprehensive mental health centers. *Am J Public Health* 54:1965, 1964.

Felix RH, Bowers RV. Mental hygiene and socio-environmental factors. *Milbank Memorial Fund Q* 26:125–47, 1948.

Fisher WH, Dorwart RA, Schlesinger M, Davidson H. Contracting between public agencies and private psychiatric inpatient facilities. *Med Care* 29(8):766–74, 1991.

Fisher WH, Dorwart RA, Schlesinger M, Epstein SS, Davidson H. Privatizing inpatient care for the seriously mentally ill: assessing the role of the general hospital. *Hosp Community Psychiatry* 43:1114–19, 1992.

Foley HA. *Community Mental Health Legislation: The Formative Process.* Lexington, MA: D.C. Heath, 1975.

Foley HA, Sharfstein SS. *Madness and Government: Who Cares for the Mentally Ill?* Washington, DC: American Psychiatric Press, 1983.

Foucault, M. *Madness and Civilization: A History of Insanity.* New York: Pantheon Books, 1965.

Fox HB, Newacheck PW. Private health insurance of chronically ill children. *Pediatrics* 85(1):50–57, 1990.

Frank RF, Salkever DS, Sharfstein SS. A new look at rising mental health insurance costs. *Health Aff (Millwood)* 10(2):116–23, 1991.

Frank RG, Kamlet MS. Economic aspects of patterns of mental health care: cost variation by setting. *Gen Hosp Psychiatry* 12:11–18, 1990.

Freiman MP. Hospital financial performance under the prospective payment system by type of admission: psychiatric vs medical/surgical. *Health Services Res* 25:785–808, 1990.

Fuchs VR. *The Health Economy.* Cambridge, MA: Harvard University Press, 1986.

Geller JL, et al. The impact of Brewster v. Dukakis on correlates of community and hospital utilization. *Am J Psychiatry* 147:988–93, 1990.

Gerstein DR, Harwood HJ (Eds). *Treating Drug Problems Vol I.* Washington, DC: National Academy Press, 1990.

Gibson RW. Private psychiatric hospitals: excellence is their watchword. *Am J Psychiatry* 135:17–21, 1978.

Gilbert N, Specht H. Foreword. In, *Social Services by Government Contract.* Wedel KR, Katz AJ, and Weick A (Eds). New York: Praeger, 1979.

Ginzberg E. The monetarization of medical care. *N Engl J Med* 310:1162–65, 1984.

Golden O. *Poor Children and Welfare Reform.* New York: Foundation for Child Development, 1991.

Goldsmith JC. Competition's impact: A report from the front. *Health Aff (Millwood)* 7(2):162–73, 1988.

Gottesfeld H. Alternatives to psychiatric hospitalization. *Mental Health Rev* 1:1–10, 1976.

Governor's Special Commission on Consolidation of Health and Human Services Institutional Facilities. *Action for Quality Care.* A plan for the consolidation of state institutions and for the provision of appropriate care services. Boston: Office of the Governor, 1991.

Greenblatt M. The future of community psychiatry: the therapeutic society. *Current Themes in Psychiatry, Vol 3.* Gaind T and Fawzy F (Eds). New York: Spectrum Publications, 1984.

Greenblatt M. Introduction. In, *Psychiatry and the Community in Nineteenth-Century America.* Caplan RB (Ed). New York: Basic Books, 1969.

Grinker RR, Spiegel JP. *War Neuroses.* Philadelphia: Blakiston, 1945.

Grob GN. The forging of mental health policy in America: World War II to new frontier. *J Hist Med Allied Sciences* 42:410–46, 1987.

Grob GN. *From Asylum to Community.* Princeton, NJ: Princeton University Press, 1991.

Grob GN. *Mental Illness and American Society, 1875–1940.* Princeton, NJ: Princeton University Press, 1983.

Grob GN. *Mental Institutions in America: Social Policy to 1875.* New York: Free Press (Macmillan), 1973.

Grob GN. *The State and the Mentally Ill: A History of Worcester State Hospital in Massachusetts, 1830–1920.* Durham, NC: University of North Carolina Press, 1966.

Group for the Advancement of Psychiatry (GAP). *Report No. 5, Public psychiatric hospitals.* April, 1948.

Group for the Advancement of Psychiatry (GAP). *Report No. 7, Statistics pertinent to psychiatry in the United States.* March, 1949.

Hadley TR, Schinnar AP, Rothbard AB, Kinosian MS. Capitation financing of public mental health services for the chronically mentally ill. *Admin Policy Mental Health* 16:201–13, 1989.

Handlin O. *Boston's Immigrants, 1790–1880.* Cambridge, MA: Belknap Press [Harvard University Press], 1941.

Holmes A. *Discourses Delivered at the Opening of the New Almshouse in Cambridge, xvii September MDCCCXVIII.* Cambridge, MA: Hilliard and Metcalf, 1818.

Horwitz SM, Stein R. Health maintenance organizations vs indemnity insurance for children with chronic illness. *Am J Diseases Children* 144:581–86,1990.

Hsiao W, Braun P, Becker E, et al. National study of RBRVS for physician services. Final report. Prepared for HCFA, Cooperative Agreement No 17C-98795/1–03. Cambridge, MA: Harvard School of Public Health, September 27, 1988.

Jarvis E. *Insanity and Idiocy in Massachusetts: Report of the Commission on Lunacy.* Boston: William White, 1855; Reprinted, Cambridge, MA: Harvard University Press, 1971.

Joint Commission on Mental Illness and Health. *Action for Mental Health.* New York: Basic Books, 1961.

Kiesler CA. Mental health policy as a field of inquiry for psychology. *Am Psychologist* 35:1066–80, 1980.

Kiesler CA, Sibulkin AE. *Mental Hospitalization: Myths and Facts about a National Crisis.* Newbury Park, CA: Sage Publications, 1987.

Kiesler CA, Simpkins CG, Morton, TL. The psychiatric inpatient treatment of children and youth in general hospitals. *Am J Community Psychiatry* 17:821–30, 1989.

Klevorick AK, McGuire TG. Monopolistic competition and consumer information: pricing in the market for psychologists' services. In, *Advances in Health Economics and Health Services Research, Vol 8.* Scheffler RM, Rossiter LF (Eds). Greenwich, CT: JAI Press, 1987, pp. 235–53.

Knapp M, Beecham J. Costing mental health services. *Psychological Medicine* 20:893–908, 1990.

Koyanagi C. *Operation Help: A Mental Health Advocate's, Guide to Medicaid.* Alexandria, VA: National Mental Health Association, 1988.

Kriegman G, Gardner R, Abse DW (Eds). *American Psychiatry: Past, Present and Future.* Charlottesville, VA: University Press of Virginia, 1975.

Lander JR. *Government and Community: England, 1450–1509.* Cambridge, MA: Harvard University Press, 1980.

Lave JR, Goldman HH. Medicare financing for mental health care. *Health Aff (Millwood)* 9(1):19–30, 1990.

Levin K. *Freud's Early Psychology of the Neuroses: A Historical Perspective.* Pittsburgh, PA: University of Pittsburgh Press, 1978.

Levine IS, Rog DJ. Mental health services for homeless mentally ill persons. *Am J Psychol* 45:963–68, 1990.

Levine M. *The History and Politics of Community Mental Health*. New York: Oxford University Press, 1981.

Levinson DF. Toward a full disclosure of referral restrictions and financial incentives by prepaid health plans. *N Engl J Med* 317:1729–31, 1987.

Levit KR, Freeland MS, Waldo DR. National health care spending trends: 1988. *Health Aff (Millwood)* 9(2):171–84, 1990.

Lewis NDC. What the war's experiences have taught us in psychiatry. In, (New York Academy of Medicine) *Medicine in the Postwar World*. New York: Columbia University Press, 1948.

Lindorff D. *Marketplace Medicine: The Rise of the For-profit Hospital Chains*. New York: Bantam Books, 1992.

Linowes D, et al. *Privatization: Toward More Effective Government*. Washington, DC: USGPO, 1989.

Lynn LE. Government executives as gamesmen; A metaphor for analyzing managerial behavior. *J Policy Analysis Management* 1(4):482–95, 1982.

Macht LB, Scherl DJ, Sharfstein S. *Neighborhood Psychiatry*. Lexington, MA: Lexington Books, 1977.

Manderscheid RW, Witkin MJ, Rosenstein MJ, Bass RD. A review of trends in mental health services. *Hosp Community Psychiatry* 35:673–74, 1984.

Marcus M, Edelson M. Priorities in community mental health programs: a theoretical formulation. *Social Psychiatry* 2(2):66–71, 1967.

Marmor TR, Schlesinger M, Smithey RW. A new look at nonprofits: health care policy in a competitive age. *Yale J Regulation* 3:313–49, 1987.

McGovern CM. *Masters of Madness*. Hanover, NH: University Press of New England, 1985.

McGuire TG. Financing and reimbursement for mental health services. In, *The Future of Mental Health Services Research*. Taube CA, Mechanic D, Hohmann AA (Eds). DHHS Pub. No. (ADM) 89–1600. Washington, DC: USGPO, 1989a, pp. 87–112.

McGuire TG. *Financing Psychotherapy*. Cambridge, MA: Ballinger, 1981.

McGuire TG. Outpatient benefits for mental health services in Medicare: alignment with the private sector? *Am Psychologist* 44:818–24, 1989b.

Mechanic, D. *Mental Health and Social Policy, 3rd Ed*. Englewood Cliffs, NJ: Prentice Hall, 1989.

Menninger WC. Psychiatric experience in the war, 1941–1946. *Am J Psychiatry* 103:577–86, 1947.

Merritt RL, Merritt AJ (Eds). *Innovation in the Public Sector*. Beverly Hills, CA: Sage Publications, 1985.

Moran AE, Freedman RI. The journey of Sylvia Frumkin: a case study for policymakers. *Hosp Community Psychiatry* 35:887–93, 1984.

Morreim EH. The new economics of medicine: special challenges for psychiatry. *J Med Philosophy* 15:97–119, 1990.

Morrissey JP, Goldman HH. Cycles of reform in the care of the chronically mentally ill. *Hosp Community Psychiatry* 35:785–93, 1984.

Morrissey JP, Goldman HH, Klerman LV. *The Enduring Asylum: Cycles of Institutional Reform at Worcester State Hospital.* New York: Grune & Stratton, 1980.

Muszynski S, Brady J, Sharfstein SS. *Coverage for Mental and Nervous Disorders.* Washington, DC: American Psychiatric Press, 1983.

Naierman N, Haskins B, Robinson G, Zook C, Wilson D. *Community Mental Health Centers: A Decade Later.* Cambridge, MA: Abt Books, 1978.

Naisbitt J, Aburdene P. *Megatrends 2000: New Directions for the 1990s.* New York: William Morrow and Co., 1990.

National Association of Private Psychiatric Hospitals. *Annual Member Survey.* 1988.

National Institute of Mental Health. Caring for people with severe mental disorders: a national plan for research to improve services. DHHS Pub No (ADM)91–1762. Washington, DC: USGPO, 1991.

National Institute of Mental Health. *Mental Health, US, 1990.* Manderscheid RW, Sonnenschein MA (Eds). DHHS Pub No (ADM)90–1708. Washington, DC: USGPO, 1990a.

National Institute of Mental Health. A national plan to improve care for severe mental disorders. Lalley TL, Hohmann AA, Windle CD, et al. (Eds). DHHS Pub No (ADM) 92–145. Washington, DC: USGPO, 1992.

National Institute of Mental Health. National Reporting Program, *Master Facility List,* 1986.

National Institute of Mental Health. *Statistical Note 193.* DHHS Pub No (ADM)90–1699. Rockville, MD: NIMH, 1990b.

National Institute of Mental Health. *The Treatment of Psychiatric Patients in General Hospitals.* Schulberg HC. DHHS Pub No (ADM) 84–1294. Washington, DC: USGPO, 1984.

Okin RL., Brewster V. Dukakis: developing community services through use of a consent decree. *Am J Psychiatry* 141:786–89, 1984.

Olfson M. General hospitals and severely mentally ill: changing patterns of diagnosis. *Am J Psychiatry* 148:727–32, 1991.

Patterson DY. Managed care: an approach to rational psychiatric treatment. *Hosp Community Psychiatry* 41:1092–95, 1990.

Pepper Commission. *A Call for Action.* Washington, DC: U.S. Bipartisan Commission on Comprehensive Health Care, September 1990.

Redick RW, Stroup A, Witkin MJ, et al. Private psychiatric hospitals, United States: 1983–84 and 1986. *Mental Health Statistical Note 191.* Rockville, MD: NIMH Division of Biometry and Epidemiology, Survey and Reports Branch, Oct 1989.

Regier DA, Bond JH, Burke JD, et al. One month prevalence of psychiatric disorders in the U.S.—based on five epidemiologic catchment area sites. *Arch Gen Psychiatry* 45:977–86, 1988.

Regier DA, Farmer ME, Rae DS, et al. Comorbidity of mental disorders with alcohol and other drug abuse. *J Am Med Assoc* 264(19):2511–18, 1990.

Renn SC, Schramm CJ, Watt J, Derzon R. The effects of ownership and system affiliation on the economic performance of hospitals. *Inquiry* 22:219–36, 1985.

Rice DP, Kelman S. Measuring comorbidity and overlap in the hospitalization cost for alcohol and drug abuse and mental illness. *Inquiry* 26:249–60, 1989.

Ridgely MS, Goldman HH. Mental health insurance, In, *Mental Health Policy in the U.S.* Rochefort DA (Ed). New York: Greenwood Press, 1989, pp. 341–61.

Ridgely MS, Goldman HH, Willenbring M. Barriers to the care of persons with dual diagnoses: organizational and financing issues. *Schizophrenia Bulletin* 16:123–32, 1990.

Rochefort DA (Ed). *Mental Health Policy in the U.S.* New York: Greenwood Press, 1989.

Rochefort DA. Policymaking cycles in mental health: critical examination of a conceptual model. *J Health Politics Policy Law* 13:129–53, 1988.

Rog DJ, Rausch HL. The psychiatric halfway house: how is it measuring up? *Community Mental Health J* 11:155–62, 1975.

Rosen G. *Madness in Society.* London: Routledge and Kegan Paul, 1968.

Rosenheck R, Massari L, Astrachan BM. The impact of DRG-based budgeting on inpatient psychiatric care in Veterans Administration medical centers. *Med Care* 28:124–34, 1990.

Rosenkrantz BG. *Public Health and the State; Changing Views in Massachusetts, 1842–1936.* Cambridge, MA: Harvard University Press, 1972.

Rothman DJ. *Conscience and Convenience.* Boston: Little, Brown & Co., 1980.

Rothman DJ. *The Discovery of the Asylum: Social Order and Disorder in the New Republic.* Boston: Little, Brown & Co., 1971.

Salit MA, Marcos LR. Have general hospitals become chronic care institutions for the mentally ill? *Am J Psychiatry* 148:892–97, 1991.

Savas ES. *Privatization: the Key to Better Government.* Chatham, NJ: Chatham House Publishers, Inc., 1987.

Saxe L, Cross T, Silverman N. Children's mental health: the gap between what we know and what we do. *Am Psychol* 43:800–807, 1988.

Scallet LJ. Paying for public mental health care: crucial questions. *Health Aff (Millwood)* 9(1):117–24, 1990.

Scheidemandel P. *The Coverage Catalogue, 2nd Ed.* Washington, DC: APA, 1989.

Schlesinger M. Striking a balance: capitation, the mentally ill and public policy. In *Paying for Services: Promises and Pitfalls of Capitation.* Mechanic D, Aiken LH (Eds). San Francisco: Jossey-Bass, 1989, pp. 97–115.

Schlesinger M, Bentkover J, Blumenthal D, Musacchio R, Willer J. The privatization of health care and physicians' perceptions of access to hospital services. *Milbank Quarterly* 65:25–58, 1987.

Schlesinger M, Cleary PD, Blumenthal D. The ownership of health facilities and clinical decisionmaking: the case of the ESRD industry. *Med Care* 27:244–58, 1989.

Schlesinger M, Dorwart RA. Ownership and mental health services. *N Engl J Med* 311:959–65, 1984.

Schlesinger M, Dorwart RA, Pulice, R. Competitive bidding and states' purchase of services: the case of mental health care in Massachusetts. *J Policy Analysis Mgmt* 5(2):245–63, 1986.

Schroeder H. States push to privatize psychiatric care. *Health Week* 6(1):2, 1992.

Sederer LI, Katz B, Manschreck TC. Inpatient psychiatry: perspectives from the general, the private, and the state hospital. *Gen Hosp Psychiatry* 6:180–90, 1984.

Shadle M, Christianson JB. The organization of mental health care delivery in HMOs. *Admin Mental Health* 15:201–25, 1988.

Shapiro S, Skinner EA, Kessler LG, et al. Utilization of health and mental health services: three epidemiological catchment area sites. *Arch Gen Psychiatry* 41:971–78, 1984.

Sharfstein SS. Utilization management: managed or mangled psychiatric care? *Am J Psychiatry* 147:965–66, 1990.

Shore MF, Cohen MD. The Robert Wood Johnson Foundation program in chronic mental illness: an overview. *Hosp Community Psychiatry* 41:1212–16, 1990.

Shore MF, Levinson H. On business and medicine. *New Engl J Med* 313:319–21, 1983.

Starr P. *The Social Transformation of American Medicine*. New York: Basic Books, 1982.

Stevens R. *In Sickness and in Wealth: American Hospitals in the Twentieth Century*. New York: Basic Books, 1989.

Stevenson G. Contributions of war experience to our knowledge of mental hygiene. *Am J Public Health* 36:1129–32, 1946.

Sunshine JH, Witkin MJ, Manderscheid RW, Atay J. Expenditures and sources of funds for mental health organizations: U.S. and each state, 1986. *Statistical Note No 193*. Washington, DC: DHHS Publ. No (ADM) 90–1699, August 1990.

Sutton SP. *Cambridge Reconsidered*. Cambridge, MA: MIT Press, 1976.

Sutton SP. *Crossroads in Psychiatry: A History of the McLean Hospital*. Washington, DC: American Psychiatric Press, 1986.

Talbott J. *The Death of the Asylum*. New York: Grune & Stratton, 1978.

Talbott JA, Sharfstein S. A proposal for future funding of chronic and episodic mental illness. *Hosp Community Psychiatry* 33:1126–30, 1986.

Taube CA, Goldman HH, Salkever D. Medicaid coverage for mental illness. *Health Aff (Millwood)* 9(1):5–18, 1990.

Taube CA, Rupp A. The effect of Medicaid on access to ambulatory mental health care for the poor and near-poor under 65. *Med Care* 24:677–86, 1986.

Test MA, Stein LI. Practical guidelines for the community treatment of markedly impaired patients. *Community Ment Health J* 12:72–82, 1976.

Tischler GL. Utilization management of mental health services by private third parties. *Am J Psychiatry* 147:967–71, 1990.

Torrey EF, Erdman K, Wolfe SM, Flynn LM. *Care of the Seriously Mentally Ill: A Rating of State Programs, 3rd Ed.* Washington, DC: Public Citizen Health Research Group, 1990.

Tuke S. *Description of the Retreat, an Institution Near York for the Insane Persons of the Society of Friends.* York, Printed for W. Alexander, London, 1813. Psychiatric Monograph Series #7 (Reprinted). London: Dawsons of Pall Mall, 1964.

Valdez RB, Ware JE, Manning WG, et al. Prepaid group practice effects on the utilization of medical services and health outcomes for children: results from a controlled trial. *Pediatrics* 83:168–80, 1989.

Vogel MJ. *The Invention of the Modern Hospital.* Chicago: University of Chicago Press, 1980.

Wain H. *A History of Preventive Medicine.* Springfield, IL: Charles C. Thomas, 1970.

Wallen J. Use of short term general hospitals by patients with psychiatric diagnoses. Hospital Studies Program, Research Note 8, NCHSR. Washington, DC: Public Health Service (86–3395), 1986.

Ward MJ. *The Snake Pit.* New York: Random House, 1946.

Weiner, RS, Woy JK, Sharfstein SS, Bass RD. CMHCs and the seed money concept: effects of terminating federal funds. *Community Ment Health J* 15:129–38, 1979.

Weithorn LA. Mental hospitalization of troublesome youth: an analysis of skyrocketing admission rates. *Stanford Law Rev* 40:773–838, 1988.

Wells KB, Manning WG, Benjamin B. Use of outpatient mental health services in HMO and fee-for-service plans. *Health Services Res* 21:452–74, 1986.

White SL, Chirikos TN. Measuring hospital competition. *Med Care* 26(3):256–62, 1988.

Wiebel RH. *The Search for Order: 1877–1920.* New York: Hill and Wang, 1967.

Windle C, Bass RD, Taube CA. PR aside: initial results from NIMH's service program evaluation studies. *Am J Community Psychology* 2(3):311–27, 1974.

Woy JR, Wasserman DB, Weiner-Pomerantz R. Community mental health centers: movement away from the model? *Community Ment Health J* 17:265–76, 1981.

Wyman M. *Dedication of the Cambridge Hospital, April 29, 1886.* Cambridge, MA: WH Wheeler, 1886.

Young D. *If Not for Profit, for What?* Lexington, MA: Lexington Books, 1983.

Zilboorg G. *A History of Medical Psychology.* New York: Norton, 1941.

Index

About the Authors

ROBERT A. DORWART is Associate Professor of Psychiatry and Public Health at Harvard Medical School and The Cambridge Hospital and Chairman of the Mental Health Policy Working Group at the Malcolm Wiener Center for Social Policy, John F. Kennedy School of Government, Harvard University.

SHERRIE S. EPSTEIN is a Research Associate at the Malcolm Wiener Center for Social Policy, John F. Kennedy School of Government, Harvard University.